100
WAYS TO
CHANGE
YOUR
LIFE

Also by Liz Moody

Healthier Together
Glow Pops

100 WAYS TO CHANGE YOUR LIFE

THE SCIENCE OF LEVELING UP HEALTH, HAPPINESS, RELATIONSHIPS & SUCCESS

LIZ MOODY

HARPER WAVE

An Imprint of HarperCollins*Publishers*

100 WAYS TO CHANGE YOUR LIFE. Copyright © 2023 by Liz Moody, Inc. All rights reserved. Printed in the United States of America. No part of this book may be used or reproduced in any manner whatsoever without written permission except in the case of brief quotations embodied in critical articles and reviews. For information, address HarperCollins Publishers, 195 Broadway, New York, NY 10007.

HarperCollins books may be purchased for educational, business, or sales promotional use. For information, please email the Special Markets Department at SPsales@harpercollins.com.

FIRST EDITION

Library of Congress Cataloging-in-Publication Data has been applied for.

ISBN 978-0-06-333371-0

23 24 25 26 27 LBC 5 4 3 2 1

To The Liz Moody Podcast *family. My favorite people to learn, laugh, and grow with. Thanks for taking this journey with me.*

CONTENTS

HOW TO INCREASE CREATIVITY

HOW TO BE MORE SUCCESSFUL

HOW TO LOVE YOURSELF

HOW TO BE HAPPIER

HOW TO MAKE AND KEEP FRIENDS

HOW TO UPLEVEL YOUR LONG-TERM RELATIONSHIPS

HOW TO MAKE YOUR GUT FEEL GREAT

HOW TO LIVE LONGER

HOW TO FEEL CALMER

My story

As a child, I was filled with existential angst. I would stay up at night fretting about the short amount of time we have on this planet and my need to make every single moment count. It was, to be honest, pretty annoying.

But I also feel lucky that, from my earliest memories, I was never satisfied with the status quo. When I was two years old, my mother was in a serious accident, the ripple effects of which impacted my whole family: she almost lost her life, my parents got divorced as a result of it, and all our worlds were forever marked by a sense of before and after. I want to be clear: I'm not glad it happened. I hate when people pitch platitudes and try to make us feel grateful for the utter garbage life throws at us. I *do* think, though, that there are always opportunities to learn and grow, even in the hardest situations. Do I wish my mom hadn't gotten on that horse that day? Yes, 100 percent. Am I going to cling to the lessons I've learned and earned the hard way? Absolutely.

That experience gave me a hyperawareness that life is both precious and unguaranteed, and that in a world of finite time, it's up to us to make each moment meaningful. The only problem? I didn't really know what that meaning should be.

Unsure of where else to find purpose and passion, the day I graduated from high school, I flew to Europe, where I backpacked for months and ended up working at a coffee shop in Amsterdam (yes, that kind of coffee shop). I was plagued with self-loathing at the time, and entangled my desire to live large with a need to be "cool" that led me to take on a party girl persona that fit like a tight, itchy sweater. For the next few years I sought satisfaction in Molly-addled dance parties in Prague, mushroom journeys in France, cocaine-fueled late nights in Buenos Aires. One day, after smoking some marijuana I'd purchased from a questionable source in Brazil, I had a seizure. I was traveling by myself at the time, and suffering from an eating disorder that I wasn't yet willing to admit to. I remember sitting in the sand, having not eaten breakfast that morning or dinner the night before, as the haze from the weed descended into an aggressive feeling of panic and hunger. I got up and made my way to a local burger joint. I was at the counter, trying to procure the food that the flashing alarms in my body were demanding, when everything went black.

That was the day I severed trust with my body. In the years that followed, I started having panic attacks. While doctors said my seizure was caused by severe undernourishment combined with sketchy weed, I was sure that it was simply my body betraying me, and if it had done so once, it was likely to do so again.

In my late twenties, I was living in London with my then boyfriend (and now husband and regular podcast fixture), Zack. Isolated from my community, devoid of the coping structures I'd built into my life, my anxiety spiraled. I started to have panic attacks on the Tube, the already-close walls of the Piccadilly line squeezing in around me as my vision tunneled. I abandoned my cart at a grocery store after the line I was waiting in made me feel trapped and the white walls and snack-stocked aisles began to tilt on their axes. I started making up excuses not to go out with Zack and our friends. My world became the size of my house, and then my room, and then my bed, where I would lie for the entirety of the day, afraid of the panic attack I'd have if I left it.

I still remember the feeling of being horizontal under the comforter with my computer propped on its side, and thinking: *I guess this is my life now. At least I have the internet. I can stream movies. I can send emails.*

There I was, the existentially ambitious child, the person who was so intent on seizing every single moment—and I couldn't even get out of bed. I wasn't living my best life. I wasn't living *any* sort of life. A layer of depression descended on top of my anxiety. Where had I gone so wrong?

I did, however, have one critical asset: years of professional experience in finding answers. I'd been working as a journalist for over a decade by then; I had started working for the local paper when I was sixteen after I secured an interview with Hootie & the Blowfish, who were playing in my small Central Valley town in California. Shortly thereafter, I pitched a column and began writing about my experience of the world on a weekly basis. My first job out of college was running an editorial team at a start-up, which later evolved into writing for publications like goop, *Marie Claire*, and *Glamour*, and, much later, into serving as the food director for leading wellness media company mindbodygreen. I'd internalized the notion that if I had questions, there were experts out there who'd spent their lives researching the exact explanations I sought.

I began emailing people I likely had no right to contact (putting into practice one of my core mantras: never be the one to say "no" to yourself, which we'll talk about later). I wrote to a Stanford neuroscientist and asked what was going on in my brain during panic attacks, and how, from a neurochemical perspective, an anxious brain differed from a calm brain. From my horizontal position, propped up on pillows with my cat curled up against me, I sent notes that crossed the thousands of miles I no longer could. I emailed registered dietitians, hormone specialists, psychiatrists, and psychologists. I dove into published research and messaged study authors with my questions. Not all of them wrote back, of course. But some of them did. And slowly, I got a sense of why I was feeling the way I was feeling, and advice on some different pathways that might help me feel different.

Because I was still daunted by the prospect of doing, well, almost anything, I decided to start with one simple change—something that felt achievable, and that didn't require leaving my house: I committed to making a green smoothie every morning. It combined many of the food recommendations I'd gathered from the registered dietitians I'd spoken to, while also incorporating the advice I'd received from a psychologist to add some type of structure or routine to my day.

Zack picked up the ingredients for me (I still wasn't ready to go to the grocery store), and the next day, I climbed out of the safety of my bed and padded downstairs. Heart pounding, I loaded the ingredients into the blender and turned it on.

And I was healed!

Just kidding. My life didn't change so dramatically that day— but it did change. I made another smoothie the next day, and then the next, and so on. Before long, it became a habit. Soon I found myself looking forward to getting out of bed in the morning. I started to drink my smoothie at the kitchen table instead of taking it back to my room. Once I was up and wandering around the house, I'd think: *I wonder if there's anything else I could do that might help me even more?* I added five minutes of meditation and, after that, a daily reading from a book that inspired me. In time, with sweaty palms, I could even take a walk around the block.

And now, years later, I'm writing this book on a plane as I travel by myself from one country to another. Since my bout with agoraphobia, I've had high-powered magazine editor jobs in New York City; I've married the man of my dreams; I've ended my apartment lease to nomadically traverse the most beautiful places in the country; I've white water rafted and summited 14,000-foot mountains; I've published two successful books; and I'm lucky enough to have the job of my dreams, hosting *The Liz Moody Podcast*. In some ways, I've taken that anxious person, trapped in her bed, and turned her into an inspiration for my weekly work. But instead of asking the world's leading minds, "How can I live *my* best life?" I get to ask for all of us.

I also learned an important lesson on my road to healing: that our best life is the culmination of every part of our mind, body, and external environment. When I didn't have relationships and community connection, my anxiety spiked, leaving me even more isolated. When I was traveling and doing drugs and partying into the night, I hadn't addressed the trauma of my childhood that had led to my constant need for stimuli and validation. When

I didn't give my body the nourishment it needed, it rebelled acutely, and terrifyingly.

It's all connected. To get the most out of every moment, we need to learn the skills to work through our past and create meaningful relationships in the present. We need to pay attention to our finances so that we have the resources to eat nourishing food and have extraordinary experiences. We need to take care of our physical health to minimize pain and discomfort, and to give ourselves the energy we need to accomplish everything we want to each day, the cognitive ability to enjoy as many moments as possible, and the longevity to feel good for years to come. We need to nurture our psychological selves so not only are we not trapped in a bed, but we *also* tap into our potential, our contentment, our gratitude, our satisfaction.

There are amazing resources out there that provide great advice on how we can transform our physical health, or shift our mindsets, or change the way we interact with the world at large. But I wanted to create a guide that not only included the most evidence-based versions of these ideas, but also helped us connect the dots between them. Our microbiomes impact our productivity. Our careers impact our hormone levels. Our sex lives impact our sense of self-worth, and that same self-worth impacts our ability to draw boundaries with our parents or ask for the raise we know we deserve.

Moreover, the pursuit of a better life shouldn't feel like punishment. It shouldn't feel like a chore, or homework, or a list of things we're missing out on. It should feel like an opening, an expansion into how it's possible to feel. It should feel easy to understand, like chatting with a really smart friend who knows all the science but is going to explain it to you in a way that won't make you fall asleep. That's where this book comes in.

This is your all-in-one resource for living *your* unique best life. I wanted to answer the question that so many of us often have when ingesting some of the amazing research we have access to these days via books, media articles, and podcasts: *That's fascinating, but what should I actually do?*

It's a question I've become known for asking in a million different ways on *The Liz Moody Podcast*: What are the best foods for our metabolic health? How does our childhood trauma show up in our adult life, and what's one thing we can do today to rewrite damaging patterns? What's the best strategy to ask for a raise, and what specific words should we use? What's the most pragmatic, actionable way to apply this advice in order to *feel* the benefits today?

And now I've taken it even further by collecting the best advice and tools from the podcast and expanding on them to make a book full of actions. These tips distill the wisdom that the world's leading experts have shared across thousands of hours of *The Liz Moody Podcast* episodes, mixed with some of my own mantras that I've found made the largest difference in my years on this planet. You'll gain an understanding of the science, and then you'll learn how to apply it in ways that will change your life. Every single tip has an associated action. Every single lesson comes with a thoughtful way to apply it and thus reap the benefits. And every single page is packed full of takeaways—my goal is for you to feel like you're getting fifty books in one.

Some of these changes are more significant than others; you might find yourself engaging in recurring plans to benefit from the science-backed ways to make more friends (see page 165), or making over your meals to be more metabolically healthy so they fuel every single cell in your body (see page 49). Some are tiny—on page 261, you'll find a breathing exercise that can change your physiology in under a minute, and on page 64, you'll learn about the two-minute trick that fights inflammation, decreases cortisol levels, and increases resilience. Some will solve problems that have stood in your way for years, whether that's chronic pain (see page 324) or an inability to stick to a workout routine (see page 20). Some will simply change your perspective on things you already do—after reading the tip on page 148, for example, you'll never see trudging through the rain with heavy groceries the same way again.

Every single tip is designed to create real change, to help you figure out your most authentic, fully-realized self, and then become that person. Because of the format (see page xix for more on that!), your path will be different from the path of anyone else who uses this book—and that's intentional. Your best life is unique to *you*. It's not your mom's best life or your best friend's best life or that celebrity you follow on Instagram's best life, and what you eat, do, and think every day should reflect that.

There are no extreme promises, and there is no bullshit; only well-researched ideas and advice from credentialed experts, distilled into approachable, accessible actions that you can take *today*. Some habits might result in instant shifts, while others might transform your life over the course of a week or a month. Some days might nudge you in a positive direction, while others might shake your entire worldview. But I promise you this: these little changes add up to a big difference. Day after day, page after page, we'll build a rock-solid foundation for a life that will make you feel vibrant, energized, calm, confident, and ready to take on whatever the world throws at you.

This is the book I wish I'd had when I was lying alone in that bed in London. This is the book I want to give to my sister, my best friends, my mom and dad, and all of my dear listeners. This is a book of action. This is a guide to your best life.

How to use this book

After interviewing hundreds of the world's leading minds, I've learned two underlying realities about living our best life: that we all have individual paths to healing and happiness, *and* that there are a select few truths about transformation that tend to apply to almost everyone. I designed this book to reflect both of these realities, and to cut through the soft promises that litter the personal growth space.

No matter what, I recommend everyone start with the first section of the book, "How to define your best life," where you'll learn how to define your goals and measure your results. After working in the wellness industry for over a decade, I've seen far too many people pursue habits, routines, and diets that they abstractly feel are "good for" them, with no sense of why. Your time, money, and energy are precious. If you're adding anything to your life, I sure as heck want you to know why that thing is worth adding.

After that, if you'd like to read the book in a linear order, from beginning to end (like, well, a normal book), you'll find value on every single page. Start with the tips that stand out to you and bookmark others to try later, or to share with that friend or family member who you know would benefit.

At the same time, I wanted to acknowledge that your needs are different from anyone else's. To make it as easy as possible to find the information you need *right now*, I've organized this book into subsections. Each one is results-focused: you'll notice there's no "how to eat" or "how to work out" section, because depending on your needs and goals, those answers will be different. Do you want a diet to give you the fuel your cells need to thrive on a day-to-day basis? Perfect, go to the "How to have more energy" section and enjoy a metabolically balanced meal. Are you contending with constipation, bloat, or other discomfort that's impacting your ability to feel your best in your body every day? Head to "How to make your gut feel great" and we'll get right to the root of that. As your life starts to transform, you might find different tips resonate more, and you can visit ones you've tried and ones you haven't time and time again.

That all said, I can hear some of you saying, "Just tell me exactly what to do!" and I get you—I've been there, too. If that's you, you can also treat the whole book as a plan, trying out every tip in order at a cadence that feels good (I recommend no more than three a week, to avoid overwhelm and better help you discern what's really working for you).

Of course, I understand that sometimes we just want inspiration; I have so many days where I feel *blech* and know that I simply want to feel better. While the book has sections that address this (I'd begin with the "How to be happier" or the "How to feel calmer" section), when I'm in that mood, I find it helpful to simply flip through the pages. It's inspiring to be reminded of the many proven ways I can make myself feel better, and often, my gut will point me in the direction of exactly what I need at that moment.

Ultimately, though, this book is now yours, and your path through it is yours as well. My job was to fill it to the brim with as much life-changing knowledge as possible; your job is to use that knowledge in the way that works for you. Keep it in the bathroom so you come out of every poop inspired. Leave it on your bedside table to prime your brain in a positive direction before you fall asleep or when you first wake up. If you want to go deeper into any topic, you'll find opportunities for more learning at the end of every section. This includes related episodes of the *The Liz Moody Podcast*, books, and other resources directly from the experts.

Picking up this book was your first and crucial step toward living a life that you love. Are you ready for the next one? Let's dive in.

HOW TO DEFINE YOUR BEST LIFE

1.

Above all, suffer less.

One of my core philosophies is that wellness is a tool, not a state or destination. It's not something that we try to *attain*; we cannot wake up and be well. Rather, it's a resource we can lean on in service of our best life. We can build our resilience to be more prepared when hard times come (see page 148); we can tackle impostor syndrome so we can achieve the success we deserve (see page 111); we can eat food that nourishes our gut so the primary bellyaches in our lives come from laughing too hard with friends.

It means, though, that the second wellness is making your life *worse*, not better, it's no longer wellness. If you're so concerned about the contents of a restaurant's menu that you miss out on a meal with your friends—you're not using the tool that is wellness to enhance your life. If you're swearing at yourself during a workout, critiquing the shape of your body, trying to hate yourself into a shape that society happens to have decided is trendy at this particular moment—that's not wellness. If your morning routine is so long that just thinking about checking off all the boxes stresses you out—well, that's not really your best life, is it?

Look, we've gotten a lot of things wrong as, you know, humans functioning in society. And while this one is not at the top of the list, it's still pretty painful to think about: somewhere, sometime, along the way, we became convinced that being well or "healthy" was often synonymous with suffering. Sometimes we lose sight of the fact that psychological suffering is as impactful as physical.

Science also supports the perspective that suffering doesn't mean success: numerous studies have shown that people will choose more nutritious options over ones that are less so when the more nutritious ones are presented in ways that emphasize their pleasurable elements.[1] The same holds true for exercise—over and over, doctors on my podcast have emphasized that the *best* workout for our health is the one we actually enjoy enough to stick to.

Shifting your mindset is the first step in changing your relationship with your healthy habits. Instead of thinking, *I have to meditate*, try to think about the *benefits* you're deriving from meditating. How do you feel after? Clearer? Calmer? More focused? Instead of hating the way your cellulite looks at the gym and pushing your limits on the weights to try to hate yourself into a body you love, focus on how strong your body feels. How do you want to use the strength you're creating for yourself? To live as long as possible, so you can be smiling at the dinner table in your nineties surrounded by people you love? To hike to a hidden alpine lake? To dance at a club until dawn? Let these things motivate you.

After shifting your mindset, the next step is shifting your actions. If you don't like the way a specific habit feels, you can almost always shift to something you *do* like that will offer similar benefits. If you find yourself dreading an activity, could you change to a different one (if you hate running, maybe explore group fitness, or try weight lifting, which to me feels like using an adult jungle gym), or could you combine it with something you *do* love so you'll look forward to it (see page 28 for more on that)? Could you find a workout buddy and use movement as your time to catch up together? Could you hike, snowshoe, or otherwise use your daily activity as an opportunity to commune with nature?

I find that healthy food in particular has a bad reputation: one of the most harmful and pervasive myths is that the flavor and appeal of healthy food are synonymous with that of cardboard. Imagine how differently we'd all approach filling our plates if we believed that garden-grown goodness not only fueled us, but also satisfied our palates! Imagine if we weren't forced to finish our veggies, but were taught to indulge in them (this was not me, by the way—I was raised largely on microwaved frozen hot dogs, just another reminder that our present success need not be defined by our childhood).

In many cases, adding nutrients to our food actually *makes* it more delicious: pound for pound, most herbs contain more antioxidants than the vegetables we typically eat, and they contain compounds like thymol[2] and carvacrol[3] that studies have found to fight inflammation, viral and bacterial infections, cancer, and more—and they make your food taste and look *way* better. I'll top my strawberry oatmeal with fresh thyme; I'll put dill in my eggs; I'll tear fresh basil leaves over my pasta. Herbs are also an amazing way of making your leftovers feel bright and fresh again, and sprinkling on a little bomb of potent therapeutic benefits at the same time. Spices, too, are packed with flavor and therapeutic benefits; I rarely make a green smoothie without including cinnamon or cardamom, and tend to double the amount of spices called for in most recipes I follow. Food—*including* nutrient-dense food—is one of the greatest pleasures in our world, and there aren't any awards for missing out on that because you think choking down an unseasoned boiled chicken breast makes you healthier. If you don't crave your food, ask yourself, what would make you *excited* about eating it?

Some suffering is an inevitable part of the human experience (for more on reframing elements of that, see page 310). Some small suffering even leads to feeling better after (see page 64, or page 148). But if you're filling your days with habits you dread or selftalk that makes you feel terrible, you're making your life worse, not better. You're increasing your net suffering, which is not an approach that's enjoyable or easy to stick to in the long run.

If you find yourself saying, "If I don't do this ten-step skincare routine, I'm going to look so old," or "I can't go out to dinner with my friends, the food at that restaurant doesn't fit into my diet," you are no longer on the path to your best life. The second that something designed to make your life better starts to stress you out or limit you, it's no longer healthy for you—*and that's okay.* That's wonderful, in fact. Because it means you're becoming more tuned in to your needs and your outcomes, and that is a nonnegotiable on any personal growth journey.

For your meals, your workouts, and the rest of your habits, ask yourself: *Is there a way I can switch my thinking to make this enjoyable? And if not, is there a way I could either modify what I'm doing or switch to something else entirely to derive both the inherent benefits of the activity and the myriad other benefits that come from that activity being pleasurable?*

2.

Do N-of-1 experiments.

One of the most frustrating, important, and underdiscussed realities of trying to be our happiest, healthiest selves is the uniqueness of each of our human bodies. We're all looking for universally applicable advice, when the truth is, we're all individual in terms of not only our biology but also our finances, our priorities, our access, our advantages or disadvantages within the systems in which we live, our relationships, and more.

I like to think of optimization advice as existing on a spectrum: some of it works for almost all people, some might work for half the population, and some might be effective for just a few people—but for those few, it could make all the difference. This is why I never dismiss people who credit something for their better health or life that perhaps doesn't have reams of research behind it, or, on the flip side, those who find that something a lot of people love or a lot of studies support makes absolutely zero difference for them. While I've made every possible effort to fill this book with tips on the more universal side of the spectrum, what works for you, what you need, and what you're interested in will make some tips more relevant than others. This is where Dr. Sara Gottfried's advice to run an N-of-1 experiment on yourself comes into play. In clinical trials, an N-of-1 experiment is a study in which the participant pool is a single individual—in this instance, you!

When I interviewed Dr. Gottfried, a Harvard-educated MD and *New York Times* bestselling author, we discussed the work of

National Geographic researcher Dan Buettner. Buettner analyzes so-called Blue Zones, areas around the world that are home to the greatest concentrations of centenarians, using epidemiologic data about their habits. But the data simply reflects the experience of a specific population within a specific environment, which can make it difficult to concretely disentangle and extrapolate what we should try at home to achieve the same results. Do people who live in the Blue Zones make it to extraordinarily old age because of their diet? Their genes? Their community? Something in the soil that we have yet to identify that impacts their microbiome? Or, more than likely, some combination of the above?

"How do we take this epidemiological data like Blue Zones and actually apply it to the individual?" asked Dr. Gottfried. "How do we personalize it? I do it with N-of-1 experiments. For instance, on a Blue Zone island in Greece called Ikaria, they drink diuretic teas made from different wild greens that they forage. I got a collection of organic teas from this island, and I started drinking some every night, and I noticed that my blood pressure came down—not significantly, but five to ten points, and that was the only thing I had changed. That kind of experimentation can be really helpful in narrowing the general recommendations to something that helps the specific person."

Dr. Will Bulsiewicz, a renowned gastroenterologist and best-selling author of *Fiber Fueled*, also hammered home the idea of personalized recommendations. "Let's pretend that you have generalized anxiety disorder and you take a probiotic," he said. "You notice that when you take this probiotic, you have an improvement in your mood. I don't care what the research says at that point, because you introduced this microbe into your personal ecosystem and are deriving a benefit. On the flip side, let's pretend that we have a probiotic that has a randomized controlled study that shows it's great for generalized anxiety disorder. You run out and grab it at the store, you take it for a month or two, and you notice no difference. Unfortunately, it's just not a fit for your personal gut microbiome—it doesn't matter what the randomized control trial said." Randomized controlled trials are one of the greatest scientific developments in history, helping us isolate variables, reduce bias, and understand on a larger scale how interventions really affect outcomes. That said, they're not without their limitations. And ultimately, in our own lives, we're most interested in how something impacts *our* individual health.

That's where N-of-1 experiments come into play.

Before you make a change, ask yourself: What are your goals? What do you hope or expect will happen? And then when you make the change, keep track of its impact. There's a lot of technology available that makes running tiny experiments on yourself easier: I regularly use my Oura Ring to measure the impact of sleeping in a cold room versus a warmer one, going to bed earlier versus later, or reading versus being on my phone, and devices like Levels, a continuous glucose monitor from a company cofounded by podcast guest Dr. Casey Means, can help you see how your blood sugar responds to different factors like macronutrients in food or types of exercise. There are WHOOP bands, smart watches, blood pressure monitors, home blood tests you can send off to labs, and more.

If you don't want to get technology involved or don't have access to it, there are plenty of other ways to measure the effects of the changes you're implementing. If you want to try something new to help with chronic bloating or stomachaches, keep a diary of your symptoms the week before you start, and then during the time you're doing something different (this works well for addressing things like burnout, anxiety, and low energy as well). If you want to try some new supplements, add them to your regimen one at a time and wait a bit before adding the next so you can connect any potential results to a specific source. Similarly, if you eliminate certain foods or food groups, track the effects of each choice to make sure you're finding the real culprit.

The N-of-1 approach also helps on a psychological level. It gives you permission to lean into solutions that work for your specific biology and to be less frustrated if something widely touted by experts or friends just doesn't work for you. It's one of the reasons I designed this book with tips you can use as needed to address the transformations you need or want to make at that particular moment in your life. While research is immensely helpful in guiding us in evidence-backed directions, at the end of the day, your body is your own, and learning to listen to (and even measure!) what it's telling you will be your greatest asset.

3.

Think about your death.

Wait, wait, before you skip this tip, let me explain: contemplating your death doesn't have to be depressing. In fact, taking time to reflect on the inevitable end of your journey Earth-side can be incredibly life-*affirming*. Moreover, the practice can help guide you toward a life that feels truly satisfying.

When I had Alua Arthur, a renowned death doula and founder of Going with Grace, on the podcast, she shared that "being around death constantly reminds me to fully feel into life—the pain, the sorrow, the crying, the grief, and all of the joy, the mystery, the awe, that moment when I look into my partner's eyes and I feel loved. It's all awe-inspiring."

According to Arthur, we don't need to abandon our lives and become death doulas to experience these benefits. She recommended taking a few minutes to think about our own death in a tangible, specific way. "Think about your funeral, your service," she said. "Who's going to be there? What are they going to say about you? What kind of life will they say that you've led?"

Dr. Julie Smith, a clinical psychologist and bestselling author of *Why Has Nobody Told Me This Before?*, seconded Arthur's belief in the affirming power of contemplating our own demise. "It's the one thing we all have in common—that none of us are getting out of this alive—but the idea that we all die at some point is not the thing to try to numb out. It's the whole reason that we can be grateful for today," she said. "And death in itself, however terrifying and horrifying it might feel, can also create meaning in living to-day. What would you do if you knew you only had twenty days to live? The things that people come up with can feel really radical, but sometimes they're the simplest things as well. It might be, 'I'd spend more time with my family,' or 'I'd go on more walks in my favorite park.'" Wouldn't it be wonderful if we just did that thing before we were actually facing our demise?

Thinking about our death allows us to differentiate between momentary discomfort—inconveniencing ourselves or others, or embarrassment—and the deep and resonant pain of a life unful-filled. Today, take a moment to contemplate your death. What can it highlight about living a life that you're proud of today? What can it teach you about shifts you need to make? How can it guide you, as Arthur said, to feel into each moment on this day a little more? "What a mystery it is even to be able to feel the floor," she marveled. "To feel cold, or wood, or carpet, or pain in that toe that I stubbed the other day."

While I'd love this book to promise immortality (and some tips certainly do tackle longevity, see page 238), the truth is that death is coming for us all. What this book can do is try to make each mo-ment as well-lived as possible, and part of that process is zooming out to realize the finiteness of those moments, so we give each the weight and the gravitas it deserves. Thinking about our eventual death is a critical step to changing our lives today. It gives us the perspective to think about what choices matter, and what we're wasting brain space on that's ultimately inconsequential. Instead of writing a script and having no idea where it's going, we're able to look at the entire movie, and shape the first half so it gets us where we want to go in the second. Life and death are intrinsically entangled, and as such it's fitting that a book about changing your life begins with contemplating the end of it. How can your death inform what a life well lived means to you?

WANT TO DIVE DEEPER?

Listen to these episodes of **The Liz Moody Podcast:**

- "How to Overcome Fear of Death (+ Genius Tips for Navigating Grief) with Alua Arthur," episode 145
- "Ask the Doctor: Longevity Edition—What to Do NOW to Look and Feel Your Best for as Long as Possible," episode 64

Explore these resources from our expert guests:

- Alua Arthur, www.goingwithgrace.com
- *Women, Food, and Hormones: A 4-Week Plan to Achieve Hormonal Balance, Lose Weight, and Feel Like Yourself Again* by Dr. Sara Gottfried, @saragottfriedmd on Instagram

HOW TO STICK TO HABITS AND ACHIEVE YOUR GOALS

4.

Figure out your "why."

If you have a habit that you just can't stick to, it might be because you're focusing too much on the "how"—what time of day to go to the gym, how long you should meditate and what type of practice you should do—and ignoring the "why."

"We tend to over-index slightly on how and under-index slightly on why," explained Daniel Pink, the five-time *New York Times* best-selling author of *The Power of Regret, Drive, To Sell Is Human*, and more. "If I say to myself, 'How am I going to get exercise today?,' just twice in a week, change that 'how' to a 'why' conversation. '*Why* am I getting exercise?' Well, because I know that I feel mentally sharp when I exercise. I know that the older I get, the more I need to stay physically fit because I want to be there for my family."

Often, our reasons for *not* doing something aren't grounded in logic; instead, it's because we haven't identified how the thing we're attempting to do aligns with our values and goals. Following the train of reason can uncover layers of motivation you might not have even known existed—and, on the flip side, can surface reasons why something might not be worth motivating yourself to do at all. If you don't know your why (I get messages constantly from people who are trying to add habits or take supplements simply because they saw someone else doing it) *or*, worse, your why comes from a negative place, motivation likely won't be easy to come by.

For years, if you had asked me why I worked out, I would have answered that I wanted my body to look a certain way. I wanted a cute butt and flat abs and long, lean legs—attributes that every magazine since I started reading had told me I should be working toward. While the pursuit of media-generated standards of "beauty" is obviously problematic in many ways, for me, it also came with a very practical downside: without the promise of an immediate reward, it was tough to stay motivated.

Our brains like immediate gratification. While some people can hit the gym every day in the name of bodily changes they *might* start to see in a few months (if they're incredibly consistent), that type of willpower isn't available to many of us. Temptation bundling (see page 28) helped me get over part of my exercise hump, but another key strategy was tuning in to the immediate rewards that came from moving my body.

After all, there are hundreds of studies that show exercise has myriad benefits for our mental and physical health, including improving our sleep,[1] cognition,[2] and mood.[3] But I was missing all those perks because I was so focused on the shape of my butt. When I consciously shifted my narrative around workouts, everything changed. Instead of lifting my shirt to check the state of my stomach, I focused my attention on the feeling of my morning brain fog clearing. I replaced thoughts about how many calories I was burning with thoughts about the anxiety dissipating from my body, or the energy permeating my cells.

Then, after my workouts, I started to tune in to how I felt and *attribute* those rewards to the workout. If I slept well, I would actively think about the sweaty workout I had done that morning; conversely, if I spent the night tossing and turning, I'd flip back through my file of the day's memories to consider how much I'd moved my body.

It also opened the door for other whys that I hadn't considered. According to Dr. Robin Berzin, founder of Parsley Health and author of *State Change*, "You can do a 10- to 20-minute workout and support your metabolism, improve cognitive blood flow, lower inflammation, sleep better that night, and start to build muscle mass."

Beyond that, "any exercise—swimming, walking, biking, hiking, sex—raises levels of endorphins in the brain, which is going to activate the release of naturally occurring opioids that can help with the reduction of pain,"[4] explained leading global pain expert and *The Pain Management Workbook* author Dr. Rachel Zoffness.

Thinking about the benefits of exercise beyond your body shape also widens the scope of what types of movement you might be inclined to try. I never enjoyed doing yoga because I didn't think it burned enough calories to be worth my time, but now I appreciate it for the many benefits it *does* offer, like stimulating my fascia,[5] or body's connective tissue, and relieving my stress,[6] which has cascading positive hormonal effects.[7]

The same philosophy applies to any new habit you're trying to integrate. You can even spend some time researching the benefits to see if they align with your actual goals. Wanting to fuel your body so you have the energy to stack your day with everything you want to do is going to be far more motivating than thinking about how your food impacts your abs. If you're trying to start a meditation habit, think about the reasons behind it (do you want to be calmer? More focused?) and pay attention to how you feel after each session. If you're adding a new supplement, make sure there's a why beyond "it's trendy right now" or "my friend/that influencer I follow takes it."

Write down a few of the habits you've struggled to integrate and consider the why behind them. Have you been trying to shame yourself into adopting new practices, filling your mind with societally-based reasons that, come to think of it, make you feel terrible about yourself? Could you change the conversation around it to come from a place of love? Write down what a different why for that habit might be; try it on to see if it feels more motivating or meaningful. If you can't figure out your why, examine whether that habit is even worth pursuing. Is there a practice that might better serve your goals? We live in a world of "shoulds," and frankly, most of us don't have time to fill our lives with habits based on other people's goals or desires. Figuring out that there's no reason at all behind the habit you're trying to adopt can be wonderfully freeing; you can create the space to fill your days with habits that actually serve your needs.

5.

Utilize the fresh start effect.

The "fresh start effect" is a little trick that makes accomplishing your goals or sticking to a new habit easier and more effective. The best part is, it doesn't take any additional effort—just a little bit of calendar finagling.

When I interviewed one of the researchers who coined the term, Dr. Katy Milkman, Wharton professor and author of *How to Change*, she explained: "We don't think about our lives linearly. Instead, we think about them as if they unfolded as a series of chapters, like we're characters in a book. One chapter might be the college years. Another might be the years working at this company, or living in that city. Every chapter break gives us a sense that we have a fresh start, a clean slate, and a new beginning. Whoever we were before that chapter break came around, you can say, 'That was the old me. The old me might have failed to achieve their goals, but the new me is going to be different and able to succeed.'"

One of the keys to making new habits stick, then, is to take advantage of these natural shedding-of-self moments, which Dr. Milkman says are actually quite predictable and common in our lives. The most famous, of course, is New Year's—there's a reason people are often inspired to set goals on the first day of January. As someone skeptical of New Year's resolutions, I was surprised to find that Dr. Milkman's research meant that setting a goal on January 1 makes us more likely to accomplish it. Essentially, we're telling ourselves that we're a different person coming into this new year than we were in the past, and that perspective shift is proven to make success more probable.[1]

But January 1 only rolls around once a year, and no one wants to wait hundreds of days to kick-start their new goals or habits. The good news? There are fresh starts *all the time*—if you know where to look for them.

"Every Monday is a fresh start—on Mondays, we see spikes in goal setting for everything from health and wellness to education to our finances," explained Dr. Milkman. "The beginning of a new month is a fresh start. The celebration of birthdays is a fresh start. There are certain holidays where we see fresh start effects; dates that we associate with new beginnings, like the start of spring or Labor Day, which kicks off that back-to-school energy." Even picking up this book is a fresh start—you're no longer the person you were before you had access to all of this information.

To take advantage of the fresh start effect, you can lean into natural fresh start moments, like the ones Dr. Milkman gave as examples, as opportunities to build new habits in your life. The you from last month might not have been good at taking care of her finances, but she's gone; it's a new month, a new chapter, and there's a higher likelihood of the new you being someone who can spend and save in ways that align with your values.

If you don't want to wait for one of those natural fresh start days to roll around, you can cheat by *creating your own fresh start*. "There's research showing when you move to a new house or engage with a new community, it gives us a fresh start sense as well," Dr. Milkman explained. If you're stuck on a project, find a new coffee shop to work at. If you can't stick to a workout routine, join a running or hiking club in your community. If you're struggling with drinking less alcohol, spend time with a group of friends who don't drink to get yourself out of the habit of bars being the go-to socialization space. Look for ways you can intentionally turn the page and start a new chapter in the book of yourself.

Whether you have a goal of your own in mind or want to turbocharge the hundreds of actions and new habits in this book, identify a fresh start moment (the beginning of a month, a new home, a Monday, a new year, a new job—the possibilities are endless) and commit to beginning your shift on that day. It's a tiny tweak, but it'll make you far more excited about—and likely to achieve—your goals.

6.

Set bite-sized milestones.

There's a common mistake we make when it comes to goal setting, and it's one of the key reasons so many of us fail to reach the targets we create for ourselves: we set a goal that's too large, or that we'll achieve too far off in the distance.

"It's critically important to define not only the long-term goal, but the bite-sized goal," explained Dr. Katy Milkman. The bite-sized goal—the smaller action you'll take *today* to move you in the direction of the larger accomplishment—is the one that many of us are often missing.

In addition to helping you define the present actions needed to get to your desired end point, setting bite-size goals can also make your goals feel less daunting. "It's not this big, global 'I want to get in shape,'" Dr. Milkman explained. "It's 'Each day I'm going to sweat. Each day I'm going to walk for ten minutes.'" It makes the goal feel less intimidating, and far more accomplishable.

Bite-sized goals also help combat procrastination. "If you're making a commitment to something you want to do on a daily basis, as opposed to just an abstract long-term goal, then you're not going to want to miss that specific daily achievement," Dr. Milkman shared. "The more you can break down that big goal into the components you need to achieve, the harder it's going to be to procrastinate, because now you're missing a specific, measurable objective, instead of saying, 'Oh, I can put it off till Friday,' or 'I can finish that next week.'"

Breaking down my larger goals into bite-sized ones has been a key component of my personal success. With the book you hold in your hands, I didn't simply say, "I want to write a book." I set a daily word count goal, and, whether I was creatively inspired or not, I hit that goal day after day. Adding one vegetable to every meal (page 199) is a bite-sized goal that has changed my life and is far more digestible (see what I did there?) and concrete than "eating healthier."

Write down one big goal you'd like to achieve, then write down a small action you're going to take on a daily or weekly basis to get there. If you want to learn a new language, maybe you commit to spending ten minutes on a language app every day. If you want to feel more connected in your relationships, maybe you commit to calling or texting one friend or family member every day. If you want to feel healthier or happier, well, there are plenty of tips in this book that you could commit to implementing daily.

7.

Use a success framework.

When I first heard that there was a science to setting goals in a way that makes us significantly more likely to achieve them, I was flabbergasted. Why weren't more people talking about this? Moreover, it turns out that many of us are actually setting goals in ways that make them *less* likely to come to fruition.

When I had her on my podcast, Dr. Samantha Boardman, a Harvard-, Cornell-, and University of Pennsylvania-trained positive psychologist and the author of *Everyday Vitality*, shared research by NYU professor Dr. Gabriele Oettingen into the science of motivation. Dr. Oettingen found that the act of imagining oneself achieving a goal actually *stands in the way* of accomplishing it.[1] The visualization gives people enough of a sense of accomplishment that they feel *less* motivated to go after the thing they want in real life. Moreover, when we positively picture completing a task, we teach our brains that the task will be easy, so in an attempt to be efficient, the brain devotes fewer resources to the task. All of a sudden, we're less motivated, with fewer resources to tackle any challenges that might arise.

That's where the WOOP method comes in. In only five minutes, you can set up a system proven to make you far more likely to achieve anything you want to accomplish.[2]

"The W stands for 'What's your wish?' Is it spending less time on your phone, or more quality time with your family?" Dr. Boardman explained. This is the first step of goal setting, the one many of us are actually good at: figuring out what we want.

"The first O stands for Outcome: What would be the outcome?" Dr. Boardman continued. Visualize what it would really be like if your wish came true. How would your life be different? Identifying the best possible outcome has two critical benefits: it provides a check to make sure that the goal is actually taking us in our desired direction, and it gives us the motivation of seeing where we'll actually end up if we achieve our goal.

The last two letters are a crucial, and often missing, part of goal setting and achievement—the O is for Obstacle, and the P is for a Plan to override it. Figuring out what internal factors might get in your way and specifically preparing for how to surmount that challenge is a key strategy of top performers across all disciplines.

What's holding you back from your wish? What's your primary inner obstacle? If your goal is regular morning gym sessions, but you always hit the snooze button, that might be your obstacle. Identifying it allows you to make a plan to overcome it—maybe you go to sleep earlier, put your alarm clock across the room so you have to get out of bed to turn it off, or switch your workout commitment to a different time of day. Or maybe the obstacle is internal: maybe you don't identify as a person who works out, or you're working out for reasons that don't truly resonate with you (see page 17). Dig deep, and don't accept excuses. Being brutally honest about your obstacle is how you'll formulate your plan, which will propel you over the hump and into the life of your dreams.

The WOOP method works because it moves beyond positive thinking and into the specifics of overcoming challenges and mapping toward achievable results. It's been shown in studies to help people increase their physical activity levels,[3] take better care of their mental well-being,[4] study better,[5] improve their social behaviors,[6] and improve time management.[7]

According to Dr. Boardman, there are benefits even beyond achieving our goals: "Closing the gap between action and intention is one of the best ways to start to mitigate sources of stress in our lives." Essentially, chronically *wanting* to do something and not doing it can cause the type of low-grade background stress that leads to burnout, health issues, and generally just feeling awful. Finding a functional way to achieve your goals is a potent, and oft-overlooked, stress-fighting technique.

I find it best to take out a piece of paper and make four horizontal rows, writing one letter in each row so that it reads "WOOP" vertically down the page. Then I fill in each row, and suddenly, I have a science-backed plan for making my dreams come true.

8.

Try temptation bundling.

A core part of making a new habit stick is making it *fun*, and let's face it: for all of us, there are some activities that are inherently *not* fun. For me, working out falls into that category. While I crave the feeling I get after a good sweat (see page 17), I find the process of exercise so miserable that it's taken me years to build a consistent practice. One of the keys to making exercise a habit has been using a tactic Dr. Katy Milkman calls temptation bundling.

"Temptation bundling is a very specific tool for making it more fun to pursue your goals," Dr. Milkman explained. She actually came upon the concept in response to the same challenge I struggled with. "When I was a graduate student, I'd come home at the end of a long day of classes, and all I wanted to do was curl up on the couch and binge watch lowbrow TV shows. My homework wasn't getting done, my exercise wasn't happening, and I was kind of a mess," she shared. "Then I set a rule for myself: I decided to only let myself indulge in the TV shows I craved if I was at the gym on the elliptical. Suddenly, at the end of a long day of classes, all I wanted to do was get on my workout machine and find out what happened next to the characters I was invested in. Time would fly while I was there, and I'd come back to my apartment feeling refreshed and completely ready to dive into my work. I'd had my break, I'd gotten my rejuvenation, and I was ready to focus. It was life-altering."

Dr. Milkman started realizing there were a lot of ways she could combine a chore that she dreaded with something that was a source of pleasure, which would make her more inclined to do the chore. "For studying, I'd only let myself pick up my favorite beverage from a favorite café when I was on the way to the library to hit the books," she said. "Or I'd save my favorite podcasts to listen to while I was folding laundry and doing dishes or meal-prepping."

Since her initial discovery in graduate school, Dr. Milkman has performed studies that show temptation bundling increases the rate at which people achieve their goals, including one where giving participants gym-only access to audiobooks led to them going 51 percent more frequently.[1] The key is to reserve the temptation—whether it's a favorite podcast, TV show, snack, or something else—for only those times when you're engaging in the less-desired activity. "Otherwise, it isn't such a temptation, and you don't necessarily build the association between these two things as strongly," Dr. Milkman said.

I now reserve my favorite podcasts to listen to when I work out, and I watch my favorite TV show while I fold laundry (a task I loathe). Your rewards may be different, and the tasks you dread might be different as well. But whatever they are, try tying them together, and see if the association is the thing that helps the habit finally stick.

WANT TO DIVE DEEPER?

Listen to this episode of The Liz Moody Podcast:

- "The Secret to Getting in Shape, Sleeping Better, Saving Money, and Being More Confident and Productive (Yes, Really!) with Dr. Katy Milkman," episode 105

Explore these resources from our expert guests:

- *How to Change: The Science of Getting from Where You Are to Where You Want to Be* by Dr. Katy Milkman, www.katymilkman.com
- *Rethinking Positive Thinking: Inside the New Science of Motivation* by Gabriele Oettingen

HOW TO
WAKE UP BETTER

9.

Take a circ walk.

If you're a part of my online community, chances are you've heard me talk about my beloved circ walks, a key part of my morning routine. "Circ" stands for "circadian," and the point of the walk is to expose my eyes to sunlight to help regulate my circadian rhythm.

Your circadian rhythm impacts your alertness during the day and the quality of your sleep at night, but its influence on health goes far beyond the sleep/wake cycle. "Almost every cell in our body, save for our red blood cells, is attuned to that circadian rhythm,"[1] explained Yale-trained MD, herbalist, and *Hormone Intelligence* author Dr. Aviva Romm. "Your liver function, your bowel function, your thyroid, your gut microbiome—it's all deeply tied to that circadian rhythm."

One of the best ways to set your circadian rhythm? Expose your eyes to light in the morning. Morning-light viewing is one of the top daily practices cited by experts on the podcast—it wakes up an area in our brain called the suprachiasmatic nucleus, or SCN, often referred to as the brain's master clock, which regulates the circadian rhythm in the body.[2] "For most of human history, we spent far more time outdoors, and we didn't have artificial light," shared Dr. Casey Means, a Stanford-trained physician and chief medical officer at metabolic health company Levels. "Seeing the sun first thing in the morning told the eyes—and therefore the brain—that it was morning. Just as food is molecular information for our cells and genes, light is energetic information for our cells and genes."

Light is so important to our circadian rhythm that small-scale studies have shown that removing ourselves from the artificial lights of modern life by going camping for just a few days can help reset our circadian clocks (it led to a 69 percent shift in circadian timing![3]) and improve sleep, a fact I keep in my back pocket for times I'm experiencing insomnia. But you don't need to take to the woods to benefit from morning-light viewing on a daily basis. The goal is simply to view sunlight as close to when you wake up, but after the sun rises, as possible, when the light is more blue in tone.

The experts I interviewed all suggested different ways to get in your light exposure. Sleep scientist Vanessa Hill eats her breakfast outside on her balcony; if the weather isn't cooperating, she'll sit right next to a window. She also drives to work without wearing her sunglasses. Dr. Means brushes her teeth outside, and if it's warm enough, she'll do her morning journaling practice in the yard.

My personal preference is to take a circ walk, or a quick walk outside as close to when I wake up as possible. I don't put on any airs for this: I toss on sweatpants, leave my hair messy, and just head outside. The walking isn't strictly necessary for the light-viewing benefits (Hill shared that sitting is more than enough to wake up your SCN), but I enjoy it and it helps me wake up (there's science behind the mind-clearing impacts of morning movement; see page 41).

The key takeaway is that our circadian rhythm matters for so much more than falling asleep and staying awake. It impacts our hormones, our gut health, our immune systems, and more. I think of my daily circ walk like taking a multivitamin—a small action that has cascading effects on whole-body health.

CIRC WALK FAQS

What is a circ walk?
A five- to thirty-minute walk outside first thing in the morning that helps regulate your circadian rhythm for the entire day.

What are the benefits?
Regulating your circadian rhythm can help with sleep, energy, productivity, regular bowel movements, gut health, hormone health, mental health, metabolic health, and more.

How long should a circ walk be?
Any amount of time is better than none. I aim for ten minutes on sunny days.

Wait, does it still work if it's not sunny out?
Yes! Just try to walk a little bit longer, around thirty minutes (you're looking for a total amount of lux to reach your eyes, and there's less lux on less sunny days). But as long as the sun is up (even if you can't see it through the cloud cover), you're getting the benefits.

What if it's dark outside when I wake up?
Wait until it's light out! You want to go outside as close to sunrise as possible.

What if I'm already at work before it's light out?
Take a quick break, if you can. When I had to commute in the dark for an office job, I used to go pick up my coffee, take a walking meeting, or just take an extended bathroom break to sneak in my circ walk.

What if I'm not able to walk?
Sitting outside works too, and being near a window inside even has some benefits, albeit fewer. The benefit is the sun in your eyes—walking is just the cherry on top.

Should I wear sunglasses?

No! You don't want to block the light entering your eyes. Wear your sunglasses the rest of the day to protect your eyes, though.

Should I wear sunscreen?

It's a short enough time period and low enough UV exposure that you should be fine without. I personally put on a quick coat of face sunscreen, but that's just because I've spent a lot of money on my skin over the years and want to protect my invest-ment. A hat is a nice compromise!

What if I wear contacts or glasses?

As long as they don't block UV rays, you're fine!

How first-thing-in-the-morning does it have to be? Can I poop first? Can I drink my coffee?

The goal is to walk as close to when you wake up and as soon after sunrise as possible—so if you wake up at nine and the sun has been up for a few hours, you want to get out as quickly as you can. But ten minutes here and there isn't going to make a difference. Make your coffee (you can take it with you on your walk!). Definitely take your poop! Just be thinking: Once the sun is up, what's the soonest I can comfortably get outside and get some light in my eyes? *You don't want to wait too long, though: try to finish your walk by 10 a.m. to really catch the sun at the right viewing levels.*

It's cold out! Can I just view the sun through a window?

Seeing any natural light is better than no natural light (if you're struggling to stay awake during the day, sitting by a window can help a lot), but you really want to be outside for the most benefits. Find yourself a great coat, and get outside!

10.

Establish a morning ritual.

Sometimes simply getting out of bed in the morning is a challenge for me. It sounds easy enough, I know, but somehow in the moment it feels nearly impossible, and I find myself wasting minutes, even hours—all of which are filled to the brim with self-flagellation— before I can finally force myself to get up. According to psychologist Dr. Julie Smith and sleep scientist Vanessa Hill, the secret to getting yourself out of bed is having something to wake up for.

We often expect that "something" to be intrinsic, meaning we're motivated to get out of bed by an inner drive. And sometimes, that's the case. "Intrinsic motivation is really powerful in helping us to do things when we don't feel like it, because we can tell ourselves that we're on the right path," Dr. Smith shared. "When I was on my book tour, I had to wake up incredibly early to go on a television show. I kept thinking, 'Why am I putting myself through this?' At that moment, I could rely on my intrinsic motivation to remind myself of why I'm doing this: there's a wider purpose and it involves me practicing what I preach and living by my values, which involves courage and doing things that I'm afraid of. Intrinsic motivations are where you say, 'It's okay. It's uncomfortable, but I'm on the right path.'"

However, those types of intrinsic motivations aren't always available to us—maybe we're working a job we're *not* excited to hop out of bed for. That's not a reason to beat ourselves up; it's the reality of many of our lives. The key, in those types of circumstances, is to bring awareness to that fact and switch to providing yourself with *extrinsic* motivation. And that's where the idea of a morning ritual comes in.

"Creating something fun for yourself to engage with in the morning is one of the best ways to get yourself out of bed," Hill explained. "I'm obsessed with coffee, so as soon as I wake up, I'm excited to go make it."

We're all going to respond differently to different rewards, but try to find something, no matter how tiny it is, that makes you feel excited to get out of bed. "Sometimes I'll get really delicious breakfast foods, so I know those are there when I wake up and I get excited to eat them," said Hill. "It could be a daily crossword, or a coffee, or going for a morning run. You just need to create some sort of incentive to get out of bed."

Of course, you also want to eliminate negative influences that make it easy to stay in bed—for many of us, our phone is the first thing we reach for the moment we awaken, and we can quickly get sucked into a scroll hole before we even have a chance to brush our teeth (check out page 43 for how you can get your phone out of your bedroom). And if you're too tired to get out of bed, you might want to examine your sleep habits and determine your chronotype (see page 39).

But all else aside, if you're looking for a powerful way to get yourself out of bed in the morning, consider employing a little treat. It's not cheating. It's not taking the easy way out. It's harnessing the power of psychology and neurobiology to shift your behavior in your desired direction.

11.

Identify your chronotype.

Waking up early is often depicted as a virtue. There's a health halo around witnessing the sunrise, as if you can't be truly healthy unless you set your alarm for 5 a.m. On the flip side, people who sleep a bit later often feel like they're lazy or that they're guilty of doing something wrong.

Well, it's bullshit.

In truth, if you're trying to force yourself to wake up early, you could be doing more harm than good. The ideal times for you to wake up and go to sleep are based on your unique chronotype, the 24-hour cycle that your individual body follows.

"Your chronotype is your tendency to be sleepy or alert at a certain time of day," explained sleep scientist Vanessa Hill. "There've been studies showing that people who had a morning chronotype made better financial decisions in the morning, and people who were evening chronotypes made better decisions in the evening."[1]

We can use our chronotypes to help us understand when we should go to bed and when we should wake up, but they can also help us pinpoint when we are the most productive, when we get our best work done, when we make our best decisions. If you have an evening chronotype, forcing yourself to wake up early is going to make your sleep quality worse and impair your ability to thrive in all areas of your life. Conversely, if you have a morning chronotype, you'll have a hard time staying up late or making good decisions in the evening hours.

The best way to figure out your sleep chronotype is to think about how you tend to function when you're free of external scheduling pressure. If, say, you went on a two-week vacation, when would you wake up? When would you go to sleep? If you could set your own work schedule, what time would you do your deep work? What time would you do your best thinking? You can also take the Munich Chronotype Questionnaire (MCTQ) or the Morningness-Eveningness Questionnaire (MEQ), both of which are easily searchable online.

Once you've figured out your chronotype, do your best to align your schedule with your natural rhythms of alertness and rest—and stop guilting yourself if your ideal schedule doesn't support a predawn wake-up.

Of course, for many of us, living in accordance with our chronotype can be tricky, if not impossible. We live in a world that's largely built around morning chronotypes, and that's not even accounting for confounding factors like children, shift work, and more.

Luckily, there are things you can do to sway your chronotype. "There are some ways that you can try to train your body to go to sleep earlier if you do have to get up early for work and you have trouble falling asleep," Hill shared. "A lot of those involve routine. Our brains thrive on a routine. Make sure that at the same time every night, you're doing things that are calming and soothing for you. Dim the lights in your house. Give your body enough time to wind down so you can fall asleep earlier."

You can also use light exposure to make your sleep-wake cycle feel easier. "Dusk light delays the clock," explained Dr. Russell Foster, the author of *Life Time* and head of the Sleep and Circadian Neuroscience Institute at the University of Oxford. "It makes us want to go to bed later and get up later. Whereas morning light advances the clock, which makes us want to get up earlier and go to bed earlier."[2] That makes regular circ walks (page 33) especially important for evening types who want to wake up and function earlier in the morning; meanwhile, walks outside at dusk can help a morning type stay up later. While the effect is fairly immediate (according to Dr. Foster, you'll notice it the following day), you need to do it consistently to have consistent results. If you want to have no effect, dusk and dawn exposure will cancel each other out, which is what happened for most of human history when we spent the vast majority of our time outside. If you can't get outside, daylight lamps or lightboxes can provide a similar effect.

The brightness of indoor light can also impact our body's biological clock. "There was a 2020 study at Monash University in Australia where people wore a clip-on meter that measured the light exposure in their homes," Hill explained. "They found that in almost half of homes, the lights were bright enough to suppress melatonin by fifty percent.[3] For a lot of people, the ceiling lights in their home can be bright enough to suppress melatonin production and some people have all of the lights on right up until they go to bed." You can either install dimmers, be conscious of when and how many lights you're turning on, or do what I do and have one set of lamps outfitted with dim orange bulbs that you turn on when you're trying to nudge the body clock toward sleep, and other lights with bright white bulbs that you use when you're trying to nudge the body clock toward wakefulness.

You can also use quick bursts of aerobic exercise as an in-the-moment way to wake up. A study conducted at CQUniversity Australia found that exercise speeds up several of the physiological processes that occur upon waking—it increases core body temperature, boosts cortisol levels (an effect known as the cortisol awakening response), and enhances blood flow to the brain.[4] All these processes help you feel awake and alert. In the study, effects were found with as little as thirty seconds of aerobic activity, making it a quick and doable way for an evening chronotype to shake off morning grogginess.

None of these tweaks will change your chronotype, but they can help you feel better if you need to live out of alignment with it. And tiny adjustments to your routine can make a huge difference: if you can't change your wake-up time or the hour you're supposed to get to work, can you schedule your deep-thinking periods at a time of day that more suits your chronotype? Matching *parts* of your schedule to your chronotype can be an effective way to take advantage of the productivity and clarity of thought benefits (see page 75 for more on matching your day to your energy levels).

Figure out your chronotype, and do what you can to lean into it. And if you've been guilting yourself for failing to wake at a certain time or doing things that otherwise contradict your natural chronotype, consider this your official backed-by-science permission to sleep in.

12.

Get your phone out of your bedroom.

Banishing your phone from your bedroom is one of those small changes that have myriad ripple effects. It eliminates stimuli that can keep you up at night, helps you make your news consumption more intentional (see page 247), reduces decision fatigue (see page 61), limits dopamine hits (see page 148), and helps you get out of bed more easily in the morning (see page 37). In fact, it's one of the top three recommendations for overall life improvement cited by all the doctors and experts I've interviewed.

Yet so many of us resist taking this step (myself included), which is why I've created a cheat sheet to help you win your own argument with yourself.

> **Excuse:** "But I use it as an alarm!"
>
> **Reality:** You can buy an alarm clock for less than $10. There are a lot of fun options these days that incorporate lights and sound to help you wake up and fall asleep. You can also set an alarm on your phone and plug it in somewhere you can hear it but can't reach it, like in the bathroom or a closet. Then you'll *have* to get out of bed to turn off your alarm, and once you're in motion, you're likely stay in motion (see page 99).

Excuse: "How will people get ahold of me when they need me?"

Reality: Most phones these days have "Do Not Disturb" modes that allow you to specify which, if any, of your contacts are exceptions to the rule, meaning your phone won't ring or buzz for anyone *but* those people. Add the people you'd want to be able to reach you in the middle of the night to the list, set your volume to loud, and plug your phone in somewhere you can hear it but can't reach it, like the hallway or a nearby bathroom, or simply across the room.

Excuse: "I scroll to fall asleep. I can't just lie there; I'll never be able to turn off my brain."

Reality: You may not be providing yourself with interesting-enough alternatives. I've bought books that have sat on my bedside table unread for months because while they might have been critically acclaimed or otherwise lauded, they simply didn't hold my attention for long. It took me years to figure out that when I'm in a reading rut, I need a quick page-turner that I might typically be too snobby to pick up. Giving myself permission to read books that I truly enjoy versus books I think I *should* enjoy has been a game changer in motivating myself to read far more often, including before bed.

If thoughts of to-do lists and work tasks race through your head at night, a bedtime brain-dump journaling session can help, as can creating a post-work ritual to create some separation from your day (see page 267). You might also try practicing Amishi Jha's in-the-moment techniques for moving your attention gently off something you're ruminating on (see page 81).

Creating a bedtime routine can also help you fall asleep quicker. "At the end of the day, our psychology isn't that different from a baby," explained sleep scientist Vanessa Hill. "You wouldn't say to a baby, 'Just fall asleep. You need more willpower'—you set up a whole sleep routine for a baby. We do all these things for babies because we know it's effective for sleep. But then we just sit there yelling at ourselves like, 'Well, why can't you just fall asleep on demand when I say you should?'" It matters less what you do specifically: you can say a prayer, read a book, change into a fluffy robe, do an elaborate skincare ritual. The key is to simply do the *same* thing, night after night, so your body begins to associate those cues with feeling sleepy.

The scrolling is just a Band-Aid. Address the root cause of the problem.

WANT TO DIVE DEEPER?

Listen to these episodes of **The Liz Moody Podcast:**

- "Genius Hacks to Fall (& Stay!) Asleep, Eliminate Morning Grogginess, Get Deep Sleep & More with Vanessa Hill," episode 158
- "How to Hack Your Circadian Rhythm to Increase Energy, Sleep Better, Improve Gut Health, Fight Jet Lag & More with Dr. Russell Foster," episode 174

Explore these resources from our expert guests:

- Vanessa Hill, @nessyhill on Instagram
- Dr. Russell Foster, *Life Time: Your Body Clock and Its Essential Roles in Good Health and Sleep*

HOW TO
HAVE MORE
ENERGY

13.

Create metabolically optimized meals.

The word "metabolism" needs a rebrand. When I was growing up, it was peppered on magazine covers promising diet tricks to "speed up your metabolism," a code phrase, like many in the '90s, for losing weight. It turns out your metabolism is far more relevant and important for your body and far *less* diet-culture-centric than the harmful headlines made it seem.

"Metabolism is how we convert food to energy in the body," said metabolic health specialist Dr. Casey Means. "There are trillions of cells in the human body, and every single one of those cells needs energy to function properly. Metabolism is what creates that energy from food. Metabolism is the power of our life."

Our metabolism, Dr. Means explained, directly impacts how we feel on a day-to-day basis. Put simply, metabolic dysfunction means that the cells in your body aren't getting the power they need, and begin to function less than optimally as a result.

Because those cells impact and make up all parts of our body, metabolic dysfunction can have an impact on all parts of our health. Think of it this way: if the cell being impacted is in the ovary, metabolic dysfunction is an underlying component of polycystic ovarian syndrome (PCOS).[1] Metabolic syndrome puts you at higher risk for depression,[2] chronic pain,[3] or migraines. It can greatly increase your risk for developing type 2 diabetes, stroke, and heart attacks,[4] and your likelihood to develop conditions like infertility,[5] erectile dysfunction,[6] and fatigue.[7] "All of these [diseases] are found at much higher rates or accelerated by people who have metabolic dysfunction, or one of the downstream consequences of that, erratic blood sugar control," said Dr. Means.

Given that metabolic dysfunction can impact so many parts of the body and affect health in so many ways, it's clearly something we want to avoid if possible. The problem? Ninety-three percent of people living in the U.S. have at least one biomarker of metabolic dysfunction.[8]

While there are many ways to begin to address this issue (*The Liz Moody Podcast* has an entire episode on the subject!), a great place to start is to look at the components of your meals. According to Dr. Means, there are five key things to think about when creating a metabolically supportive plate: maximize micronutrients and antioxidants, maximize fiber, maximize omega-3s, maximize probiotics, and minimize refined grains and sugars.

When you eat a meal, look at the components. Is there a way to add some seeds or herbs to increase the micronutrients? (For far more ideas for micronutrient maximization, see page 226.) Could you add some fermented hot sauce, kimchi, or sauerkraut to increase the bacterial sources? (If you haven't yet had kimchi with your scrambled eggs, it's a must-try, and I put fermented hot sauce, which I buy at my local farmers' market, on *everything*.) Could you add fiber in the form of veggies, seeds, or whole grains? For omega-3s, Dr. Means loves canned sardines and mackerel, or plant-based upstream sources of omegas like chia, basil seeds, flaxseeds, and walnuts (if you are consuming plant-based omegas, just be aware that they're less bioavailable).[9]

This is by no means meant to be dogmatic—is every meal I eat metabolically healthy? Absolutely not. Are there also social, economic, and environmental factors at play that prevent people from having access to all the components of a metabolically healthy meal? Absolutely, and systemic change needs to be at the forefront of our minds alongside our individual onus. Instead of treating it as a rule, I use it, when possible, as a reminder to make valuable additions to my plate.

The next time you eat, go through a mental checklist of the five components and see what you can add to your meal to hit as many of them as possible. It'll benefit your metabolic health and likely, as a bonus, make your meal that much more delicious, complex, and satisfying.

14.

Do micro-workouts for mega-benefits.

While traditionally structured workouts offer myriad benefits (see pages 17 and 95 for more on that), an interesting and far less discussed concept kept surfacing in my conversations with experts: micro-workouts. Over and over, doctors and top performers I interviewed spoke about the power of moving in tiny bursts throughout the day, either in addition to or instead of doing a longer workout all at once.

Acclaimed physician, BBC star, and bestselling author Dr. Rangan Chatterjee has done a five-minute workout every single morning for the past three years. "I haven't missed a day, not because I'm more motivated than anyone else, but because I understand human behavior. When we're talking about the ideal form of exercise to do, I could tell you all the benefits of walking, strength training, or cardio. But if you're not going to do it, it doesn't really matter. You've got to make it easy if you want something to stick in the long term, and you really want to stack that new behavior onto an existing habit."

Dr. Chatterjee stacks his five-minute workouts onto his coffee routine: "I weigh my coffee grounds out, pour the boiling water on, and put a timer on for five minutes. In those five minutes, I either do a body-weight workout or one with a kettlebell in the kitchen. I do it in my pajamas. I don't get changed. I make it so easy."

Stanford epigeneticist Dr. Lucia Aronica does pull-ups while she's making her coffee (apparently, it's a very popular time to sneak in a workout!) and push-ups while she's making her dinner. It's far, far better to use your muscles for five minutes every single day than to plan for an hour-long workout that you never actually do.

Beyond simply being able to stick to a routine, research shows that brief periods of movement are enough to experience real benefits. "If you move even for very short periods of time, multiple times per day, you'll have better glucose and insulin levels than if you just do one chunk, even if it's the same amount of time cumulatively," explained metabolic health specialist Dr. Casey Means. In one study, researchers compared the effects of (1) sedentary behavior to (2) sedentary behavior plus one hour of morning exercise to (3) sedentary behavior with twelve hourly, five-minute bouts of exercise. Despite everyone but the sedentary group doing the same amount of total movement, results showed that the five-minute bouts of exercise had better effects on blood sugar and insulin levels.[1]

One of the best ways to sneak in these micro-workouts is to look for what positive psychologist Dr. Samantha Boardman calls "incidental ambulation" opportunities, or naturally built-in pockets of time where we can avail ourselves of movement—taking the stairs instead of the elevator, parking in the spot farthest from the store entrance, delivering a message to an officemate in person rather than over Slack.

"We wrongly assume it is going to take our energy, but it has the opposite effect. Walking is an energy-giver," said Dr. Boardman. "It reliably lifts our spirits when we're feeling down. The increase in blood and energy flow is as good for our brains as it is for our bodies." Since our conversation, I've heard her voice in the back of my head throughout my days. I park farther away, I avoid escalators and elevators, and if I'm running errands, I walk instead of drive whenever possible.

Micro-workouts also provide the enormous additional benefit of breaking up periods of prolonged inactivity throughout the day. Being sedentary for long periods has been associated with a higher risk of diabetes, cardiovascular disease, depression, anxiety, and certain types of cancer; back and neck pain; poorer metabolic health; and lower energy levels.[2] Micro-workouts disrupt that sedentariness, mitigating those negative outcomes. If you're sitting all day and throwing in a thirty-minute or one-hour workout here and there, you might be getting stronger, but your body is still experiencing the consequences of being static for the other ten waking hours of your day. While I still do my regular longer workouts, I view micro-workouts as an even more nonnegotiable part of my routine. Were I to skip one or the other, it would be the longer session.

How can you facilitate more movement throughout your day? Would it feel good to habit stack a quick workout session with an existing routine, like Dr. Aronica and Dr. Chatterjee do? Could you schedule five minutes into your calendar once an hour to take a walk, whether just around your office or outside? Could you look for opportunities to take the stairs, or walk twice as far to get to a store entrance? Pace on a call. Drink enough water, so you have to get up to pee. Your brain and your body will thank you.

15.

Establish (and stick to) better boundaries.

To say I'm not great at confrontation is an understatement. But when I talked to Melissa Urban, author of the *New York Times* bestselling *Book of Boundaries*, she made a strong case that setting boundaries is a foundational and life-transforming skill.

"When you start a boundary practice, you realize that you don't have to walk around in your relationships and in your day feeling resentful, angry, anxious, or frustrated, dreading certain interactions and avoiding certain people," Urban said. "There's so much energetic expenditure that goes along with the avoidance. Setting a boundary can be uncomfortable, but it's a momentary discomfort that leads to actual change and brings real freedom into your life. Relationships are better. You feel more trusting and open. You reclaim your energy, time, capacity, money, and physical space. You reaffirm that you are worthy of having needs and having those needs be respected."

Facing the small, momentary discomfort of establishing a boundary helps us avoid exponentially more discomfort down the line, yet so many of us avoid doing so, sending tiny yet powerful and additive signals to our brains that our desires aren't worthy of respecting. We begin to resent people for not catering to our needs—we're going out of *our* way for *their* needs, after all!—when in truth, we've never communicated what those needs actually are.

Setting proper boundaries is a crucial part of giving people the tools they need to build a high-quality relationship with us. It's not a limitation; it's a gift. If people can't or won't use those tools, that's on them, and perhaps something that will require subsequent situational adjustments on our end. But giving them the tools and expressing the needs in the first place? *That's* in our control. That's on us.

To figure out which areas might benefit from a boundary, Urban recommended exploring the places in your life where you feel some unease. "If you feel a sense of dread or anxiety, that is the very first alarm bell that a boundary is needed around a certain conversation topic or with a person. If you feel like you can't show up as your full self with somebody in a particular relationship, if you don't know where you stand with them, if you leave interactions feeling less good about yourself, or if you leave interactions and you're running through the stuff in your head of what you could have said or done—those are all giant alarm bells that a boundary is needed," she said.

In our podcast conversation, Urban shared dozens of situations in which to set boundaries and ways to set them, but one of my favorites was to take a pause before replying to anyone's invitation or request. If your boss asks you to add another project to your already full plate, take a pause. Maybe that moment gives you long enough to think through if you really have time to do more, or what deadlines would truly make sense, or frame a question about what the order of your priorities should look like. If your friend invites you to a party, take a pause. Are you excited to spend time with them in that way? Are you going to regret adding this to your calendar later? Is there another way you'd prefer to spend time with them? If your parent asks you to spend the holidays with them, or someone in your playgroup asks you to watch their child, or your partner asks you to run an errand for them—take a pause. The goal is to simply practice checking in with yourself first before you attend to someone else's needs and asking what your own needs and capacities are. It's a moment where you reinforce to your brain that *your* goals and desires factor into the equation.

"Don't reply based on what you think the other person wants to hear," Urban said. "Reply based on what *you* want and need. Maybe that want and need is that it would feel good to make this person happy, *and* that would be restorative and fill your cup. That's great! But don't do something *just* because someone wants you to." Taking the pause gives you the time you need to differentiate between the two.

And if after the pause, your answer is no, that's a full sentence.

"We've been conditioned to believe that we have to have a good reason for basically anything we want, and we've been conditioned to think the other person has to agree with or approve our reason for it to be considered valid," shared Urban. This could look like "I'm not drinking because I have to wake up really early," or "I can't come to that dinner because it's out of my budget." While you're welcome to share the reasoning behind your decisions, often it can invite problem-solving or pushback instead of the acceptance you're seeking. "We can make it an early night," your friends might say, or "We can skip appetizers and order really cheaply!"

"It's incredibly empowering just to say, 'No, thank you,'" Urban said. If someone sits there waiting for you to expound on your answer, you can sit there, too, silently sending the message that no other explanation or defense is needed. If someone explicitly asks you for a reason or pushes back on your "no," you can reinforce the original boundary: "My answer is simply no at the moment, and I'd appreciate it if you'd respect that."

If this feels scary, you can practice saying "no" with people who feel safer to you as a way to become familiar with the sensations. This builds acceptance of the idea that you can disappoint people and it is okay and, in fact, preferable to the other option—disappointing yourself. On the flip side, if you're constantly practicing pushing your own needs aside to make space for other people's—well, guess what skill you're developing? "The alternative," said Urban, "is that you give in to make the other person comfortable and you sell yourself out. And then you've given yourself the message that you are not worth holding on to your needs, that your needs are not worthy. That's a really powerful message to internalize." Your boundary muscles might be shaky at first, and that's normal and natural. You haven't been exercising them regularly!

You can also create boundaries and pauses with your actions, whether by turning off the notifications on your work email or responding to texts at a time that feels good for you rather than when the ping comes through. Identify the areas in your life that could use better boundaries, and the next time someone makes a request of you, take a pause. Your answer might be no, or you might have a counter request. And it might still be yes, but it'll be a yes that feels truer, easier, and more respectful of your needs and yourself.

16.

Activate your body's natural glucose sponges.

If you see me doing squats outside of a restaurant, well, there's a science-backed reason for it. There's nothing I love more than a small health hack that leads to big results, and activating your muscles to soak up glucose is high on that list.

When your glucose level rises sharply, your body releases a bunch of insulin in response, creating a state called reactive hypoglycemia. You might be more familiar with the term, and the feeling, of a blood sugar "crash"—it can make us feel anxious, tired, shaky, and even crave more sweets, perpetuating the cycle (so tricky and annoying). Metabolic dysfunction can lead to poor glucose control,[1] meaning more spikes and crashes, but poor glucose control (i.e., more spikes and crashes from food and lifestyle choices) can be one of the elements that cause metabolic dysfunction[2] (which can be a contributing factor for myriad diseases from anxiety to cancer; see page 49 for more)—it's a two-way street. Either way, the goal is to avoid those spikes and crashes.

A number of factors cause glucose spikes, including eating high-glucose foods (like white rice or grains, or sugar-rich foods, especially unaccompanied by fat, fiber, and/or protein, which slow down glucose absorption and elongate the blood sugar curve), eating a lot of food at once, and even experiencing stress. "When you have an acute stressor, the body will get flooded with stress hormones. It does that for an adaptive purpose—it assumes that a stressful event must mean a threat is looming, which means that you probably need to run," explained metabolic health expert Dr. Casey Means. "There's stored glucose in the liver for moments like this, so the stress hormones cause the liver to dump that glucose in the bloodstream to feed the muscles so you can escape the threat." Of course, if we're just giving a presentation or dealing with an overwhelming to-do list, we don't actually *need* to run, so the glucose simply floods our system.

But regardless of whether your glucose spike is coming from stress or a doughnut, one way to minimize the impact is by engaging your muscles to help burn off some of that glucose. "Our muscles are one of our most energy-hungry organs," Dr. Means said. "I think of them as a sponge for glucose. If you're walking, you're activating so many muscle groups, all of which will use glucose." It's also a reason to build more muscle. The more muscle you have, she explained, the more glucose your body is able to dispose of— even without additional movement.

Activating your glucose sponges comes down to a two-step process: First, incorporate resistance training or other muscle-building activity into your workouts. Second, the next time you eat food that's less glucose-friendly *or* you experience stress, activate your muscles briefly. Do twenty squats. Use it as an excuse to take a lovely stroll after a big meal (even two minutes of walking post-meal has been shown to help![3]). Any muscle activation will soak up that glucose, which will help you feel better both in the moment and in the long term.

17.

Eliminate sources of decision fatigue.

While it's hard to measure exactly how many decisions the average adult makes on an average day, some research puts the number at a whopping thirty-five thousand. That might seem crazy, until you start to add up the decisions that start the second you open your eyes: *Should I snooze? Should I get up? What should I eat for breakfast? What should I wear?* Then there are the hundreds of decisions you make at work, and hundreds more in your interpersonal relationships. It's no wonder that by the time we get home, we're exhausted. If you've ever scrolled through a streaming platform for an hour, unable to make a choice as simple as what TV show or movie to turn on, you've experienced decision fatigue.

Many of the top performers I've interviewed cite eliminating as many sources of decision fatigue as possible as one of the secrets to their success. They share stories about creating a work "uniform," like Steve Jobs's famous jeans-and-black-turtleneck combo, or eating the same thing for dinner every night. "We tend to go with a path of least resistance in general, which can be great when there's a solution that involves creating a default so you don't have to think about it anymore," explained famed behavioral scientist Dr. Katy Milkman.

Our money habits are one of the best places to eliminate sources of decision fatigue. "A lot of the best hacks that are the most useful allow you to basically put savings on autopilot," explained Dr. Milkman. It sounds simple, but even the conscious decision of deciding how much to save each month and remembering to take it out of your account—these are opportunities to experience decision fatigue or forget, so you don't end up creating the habit you want.

I Will Teach You to Be Rich author Ramit Sethi takes it a step further and recommends autopaying bills (if you have debt or can't afford the full amount, just do the minimum; it will help you avoid late fees and increase your credit score) and autopaying into your Roth IRA, if you can swing it. He even recommends taking note of big-ticket items in your future—let's say, a wedding you know you'll be attending next summer, or a trip you want to take in the fall—and working out how much you need to save each month to hit those goals, then automatically deducting that amount.

Take an inventory of your finances and see what opportunities you have to create automatic systems that make your desired goals something you don't even need to think about. You can also expand these systems to other facets of your life: Are there weekly groceries it would make sense to auto-order? A monthly toilet paper, paper towel, and cleaning supply shipment you could set up? Off-loading the cognitive processes behind these menial tasks will not only free up brain space and time to do the things you love, but, since a computer is handling it, they won't be forgotten or deprioritized.

One of Sethi's best tricks for eliminating decision fatigue is to make money rules—essentially, he automates his discretionary spending by creating categories so he doesn't waste time thinking about a purchase, because it's something that he can always afford and that he's preemptively decided provides him with enough value for the price. Books are on Sethi's list; when he sees a book he's interested in, he doesn't hem and haw and debate whether it's worth adding to his library. Instead, he simply buys it.

Eliminating decision fatigue can also include making practical changes to your environment. Instead of debating whether you should check your social media accounts before you get out of bed in the morning, you could simply charge your phone in another room. If you're trying to cut back on ultra-processed foods, instead of staring at your stash of chips and candy each night and agonizing over whether you should have some, you could choose to only keep fresh, whole-food snacks in your house.

The key is to make a decision *one time* to avoid the mental drain—and accompanying less-than-ideal results—of having to make a decision daily. Today, pick one source of decision fatigue in your life and commit to a rule designed to eliminate that decision. Spend the time to make the best decision you can now so you can reap the rewards in the future.

18.

Take a cold shower.

If I told you that you could change your life in just a few minutes a day, would you do it? That's how I view my cold shower: as one of the smallest amounts of time you can spend that still results in huge psychological and physiological changes.

Cold showers or cold plunges have been recommended by a number of the world-class doctors on the podcast, including dopamine researcher Dr. Anna Lembke, hormone expert Dr. Aviva Romm, neuroscientist Dr. Tara Swart Bieber, and metabolic health specialist Dr. Casey Means (an impressive fan club, if I've ever seen one).

Cold exposure is an example of a phenomenon called hormesis, in which a small amount of tolerable stress has a positive effect on the body. The return to the baseline of room temperature provides evidence to your body and brain about your resilience. Cold exposure therapies have been found to reduce muscle soreness and increase muscle recovery,[1] change metabolism in positive ways,[2] and fight inflammation.[3] They can also reduce cortisol levels and increase norepinephrine,[4] both of which serve to decrease stress and increase a feeling of overall well-being.

Research around cold exposure is still in its nascent phases, and we're regularly finding out more and more about the positive benefits, but the findings so far are clear: if you're looking for a quick way to inject a dose of mental and physical health into your day, cold exposure is well worth considering.

I'm not gonna lie—it took me a while to warm up to this one (see what I did there?). I'm not in a situation where I can have one of the fancy cold-plunge pools (if *you* are, you're living my dream!), but ending my daily shower with two minutes of cold water is one of my favorite health practices. I shower as usual, then turn the dial as cold as it can possibly go. I slowly count to 120 in increments of 10 (see the FAQs below for more on why), turning in every direction so the cold hits my face, the back of my neck, and my armpits.

While it's hard for me to measure some of the greater effects of my cold showers in terms of dopamine balance or metabolic health (especially when so many factors are at play), one of the reasons I've been able to stick to them for so long is the immediate difference I feel afterward (which makes sense—habits are far more likely to stick if they're partnered with immediate reward, per page 28). I'm practically roaring with energy. Any fogginess from waking up is completely eliminated. If I can let icy water prickle my vulnerable naked body—well, I can do *anything.* I take that invincibility with me throughout my day, and the sense of power shapes every interaction I have.

There also aren't that many things that offer such huge rewards in so little time—all you need are two minutes. During your next shower, lather up, rinse off, and proceed as usual—and then right at the end, turn the dial as cold as the shower can go and grit your teeth as the seconds fly by. Those few minutes might just change your life.

COLD EXPOSURE FAQS

What's the best time of day to take a cold shower?
There's not a single best time of day; you can, however, get those last 2 percent, cherry-on-top benefits by varying the time based on your goals. A cold shower after a workout will better help reduce muscle inflammation and soreness; a cold shower in the morning will promote alertness; a cold shower before bed can drop your body temperature and promote sleep. Because I add my cold shower to my regular shower, I simply do it in the morning after my workout, which makes it a sustainable habit I can stick with.

How cold does the water need to be to be effective?
Most experts that I've talked to suggested that below 58°F is ideal, with different benefits evidencing at different temperatures (and there's research to suggest that mood-boosting benefits start at as warm as 68°F[5]). I just turn my shower to the coldest it can get! There's no need for extreme cold—you should be a little uncomfortable (that's part of what's creating the benefits), but in no way in pain or physical distress.

Can I take a hot shower first or does it need to be cold the whole time?
You can absolutely take your normal shower with hot water first!

Can I go *back* to hot to warm up after the cold shower?
You get far more benefits if you let your body temperature naturally rise back to baseline. Try to end on cold.

I've seen a lot of fancy cold-plunge pools. Do I need one of those?
Cold-plunge pools keep the water temperature measurable and stable, and allow you to fully submerge your body. However,

you can experience the vast majority of the same benefits with a cold shower, which is likely free and already available in your home. Start there, and if you love cold plunging and your budget allows, upgrade later.

What if my shower doesn't get cold enough?
Again, it doesn't need to get as cold as you think (see question above). But, if your shower only gets tepid at best, you can create a DIY cold plunge: run a cold bath and add ice to cool it further, or just use a tub outside, weather and region dependent.

How long do I need to cold shower for?
Most of the benefits seem to be experienced starting at one minute under cold water, and they seem to top out around five minutes.[6] Start with one minute, and when you're able to be consistent with that, add more time in fifteen-second increments until you find your happy place.

It's so, so, so miserable. How do I make it easier?
Doing a breathwork practice (see page 261) can help—calming yourself in the middle of a cold immersion can provide good training for calming yourself in other moments of acute stress. I also like to count in chunks of ten—I feel like I can always do another ten seconds (it's only ten seconds!), and soon enough I've done it twelve times and it's over. I also find it helpful to remind myself that the difficulty of the task is part of why it's beneficial. If I can do this hard thing, taking on the rest of my day somehow seems much easier (see page 148). Singing along to one of your favorite songs can be a great way to tell time and to stimulate your vagus nerve, which will help you feel calmer.

WANT TO DIVE DEEPER?

Listen to these episodes of **The Liz Moody Podcast:**

- "Ask the Doctor: Metabolism Edition—How Your Blood Sugar Impacts Weight, Hormones, Disease & More + How to Optimize It with Dr. Casey Means," episode 150

- "Ask the Doctor: Diet and Weight Loss Myths Edition—Cutting Through Misinformation to Get to the True Science of Weight," episode 67

- "Set Better Boundaries: Overcome Uncomfortable Conversations, Spot Manipulation Red Flags & Take Back Control of Your Time with Melissa Urban," episode 139

Explore these resources from our expert guests:

- Dr. Casey Means, @drcaseyskitchen on Instagram

- Dr. Rangan Chatterjee, *Happy Mind, Happy Life: The New Science of Mental Well-Being*; the *Feel Better, Live More* podcast

- Melissa Urban, *The Book of Boundaries: Set the Limits That Will Set You Free*, www.melissau.com

HOW TO
BE MORE
PRODUCTIVE

19.

Create a rule of three.

When I met Chris Bailey, bestselling author of *The Productivity Project* and *How to Calm Your Mind*, I was expecting someone obsessed with metrics and accomplishments, someone who had an almost frenetic energy of having to get things done.

What I got was the exact opposite.

From Bailey's perspective, productivity is about making the space to do *less*, freeing yourself from mindless busyness and cultivating an intentional and deliberate life. There's a difference between being busy and being productive—we've all had days when we felt rushed and harried, but when they're over, we wonder what we've actually accomplished. A productive day is one where the ball has been moved forward in some way and progress has been made toward some sort of goal. The problem? If we're not laser-focused on being productive, the busy has a way of dominating: We clean the house but never reorganize or declutter it to keep it from getting as messy in the first place. We send a million emails but don't start the project that will change our lives. (Email is one of the greatest culprits in the busy-versus-productive sphere; many of the top performers I've interviewed limit email to specific windows during the day and stick to a strict no-checking policy otherwise.)

This is where the rule of three, one of Bailey's core practices, comes in.

"At the start of the day, fast-forward to the end of the day in your head and ask yourself, 'What three main things will I want to have accomplished?'" Bailey said. Those three things are what you should devote your focus to.

Bailey's rule of three allows you to step outside the demands of the busy, and ask yourself: *What does productivity look like for me on this day?* It pushes us to make sure we accomplish the things that are pushing our lives in the direction we want it to go. And since it's only three things, that direction feels more attainable, and there's still room for the other, less pivotal tasks that we need to do as humans on this planet. Yes, on many days, you can (and often will!) end up doing more than three things. But by intentionally starting by choosing your top three, you're always moving your life in the direction *you* want it to go. You've suddenly got a map and a trail to the mountain vista you want to see, rather than running aimlessly in one direction and then another until you're panting, exhausted, and frankly not far from where you began.

While the rule of three was initially designed for daily use, it can be utilized on a weekly, monthly, or even annual basis as well. What three things do you want to accomplish this quarter? This year? In this lifetime? Simply creating a sense of awareness around your goals can be hugely helpful in propelling you from the churn of the quotidian to the path of a far more intentionally lived life.

Write down the three things that, at the end of the day, you'll feel best having accomplished. Below that, feel free to brain dump all the other tasks occupying your mental space. If you finish your top three—amazing! Move on to the tasks below. If the exercise feels good, try it for the week, the month, the year, maybe even the next ten years. In a decade, what three things will you feel best knowing you've accomplished? Zooming out on your future can provide valuable insights into what you should spend your moments on today.

20.

Recognize the value of your time.

While all our financial dreams will differ (see page 101), most of us agree that our time is one of the most precious and limited resources at our disposal. To that end, one thing that many of the top performers that I interviewed have in common is outsourcing. "Well, sure," you might say. "They're rich: of course they can afford to hire people to clean their homes and do their taxes and make their food."

And while, yes, outsourcing is a privilege, it's available to more of us than we credit. Zack and I first hired a cleaning person when we were in our twenties, at a time when we could barely afford to eat out at restaurants and travel meant staying in a twenty-bed dorm at a hostel. But our number one fight was about the messiness of our house, and for us, the amount we spent on having someone come in and clean once a month was far outweighed by the reduction in friction in our relationship (we joked that it was like paying for couples therapy, but honestly, the impact was not far off).

Recently, I began hiring someone to prepare healthy meals for me on a weekly basis. It felt ridiculously self-indulgent at first—who did I think I was, Oprah? But during an incredibly busy time in my professional life, I took the plunge, and the *joy* I felt opening the fridge to find it full of nutrient-dense, delicious meals was *unsurpassed*. I commented on my supreme satisfaction every single time I sat down to a homemade (but not by me!) meal; I told Zack how much lower my anxiety was after taking the stress of feeding myself (and feeding myself well) off my plate. "I've never seen you this happy about *anything* you've bought," Zack said, and I realized that was true. I've had to cut down on my clothing purchases to make paying for meal prep fit into my budget, but my resulting happiness isn't even comparable. My gut feels better, my energy is higher, I'm calmer, and I have more time to devote to projects and people I love. And honestly? Because I'm never frantically ordering takeout after realizing that it's 8 p.m. and I haven't even thought about dinner, the total amount I'm spending to feed myself isn't that much higher than it was before I was paying for meal prep.

Our time is one of our most precious resources, and there are more creative ways to start to get some of it back than there might appear at first glance. A friend of mine shares a nanny with a group of friends. Another pays for someone to spend five hours a week doing errand-type tasks: returning packages, tidying the house, buying groceries. "Simply eliminating the burden of trying to remember all those tasks and figure out where to fit them into my schedule has been a game changer," she said.

If your budget permits, ask yourself if it might be possible to outsource tasks that are taking up an inordinate amount of your physical or mental energy. And before you summarily say that your budget *doesn't* allow for it (which I wholeheartedly recognize is true for some people, albeit far fewer than the number who have the initial reaction), I'd ask you to consider if the other ways you're spending your discretionary money are giving you the same joy you might derive from outsourcing. Truly picture your life with a clean house, a stocked fridge, a child-free moment to go for a walk with a friend or read a book or lie with your eyes closed. For me, that joy far, far surpasses any physical item I could spend my money on. Give your time the same value you give your closet or your electronics or whatever social media and magazines are telling you that you need to feel satisfied. Our moments are our most valuable assets; spend them accordingly.

21.

Map your day to your energy.

We all have different chronological clocks (see page 39), different brains, and different bodies, yet for the most part, we all mostly stick to the same schedule. According to career and business coach Amina AlTai, one of the secrets to getting more done *and* feeling good as you're doing it is to design your work based on your energy.

"I do my best writing and thinking at the top of the week. That's when my brain is sharpest and clearest. So, Mondays, I write and engage with bigger-picture thinking," she said. "By Friday, I really don't have capacity for any good thinking, so that's my admin day."

AlTai said we could all benefit from asking ourselves: When do we do our best creative work? When do we do our best thinking work? When do we do our best group work? Are there ways that you can design your workweek around that? "It isn't always possible inside of somebody else's organization," AlTai said. "But what's the smallest possible way that you could start to shift the parts that *are* within your power?"

Start to pay attention and even note when you're feeling particularly creative and juicy, or when you prefer to be alone versus in groups. Are there times you love being on calls? Are there times you especially hate it?

Once you start to get a picture, as much as possible, map your day to that. Maybe you schedule a deep work period during that hour between 11 a.m. and noon when you always feel most creatively inspired. Maybe you draw a boundary with yourself that you'll only check emails after 4 p.m., when your mind is worn out and can only handle admin-type tasks. You can even express your needs to a higher-up—if, for example, you have a boss who always wants to touch base in the morning, but you feel like a zombie before 10 a.m., you can tell them! In this situation, AlTai recommends what's called the SBI (Situation, Behavior, Impact) model.

"I love this framework because I think it gives us a very linear, pragmatic way to have a scary conversation," she said. First, you describe the situation ("I'd love to discuss our ten-a.m. touch-bases") and the behavior ("I'm regularly asked to show up and be able to think on my feet at ten, which isn't when my brain works best"). Then, you share the impact ("I'm stressed that I'm not performing my best in our meetings and I wish I could bring my most creative, problem-solving brain to the table"). AlTai also recommends adding a proposed solution ("Are there any other available times in your calendar later in the day?"). Your boss likely wants you to be able to feel and perform your best; they simply might be lacking the tools to help contribute to that.

Once you identify your peak times for different types of work, do anything within your power to maximize that type of work in that particular time. That might mean minimizing distractions by putting your phone on airplane mode or in another room, or it might mean taking a walk beforehand because you know you always feel more clearheaded and inspired after. "If you feel like when you're doing your creative work, you need to be in an environment where people are buzzing and there's energy there, can you then go to a coffee shop to do that thing or be in a coworking space to do that thing?" AlTai asked.

The trick is recognizing that your best work—the environment, the time of day, the outputs—won't look the same as another person's best work, and that's *normal*. By strategically identifying and nurturing those differences, you enable yourself to feel more effective, productive, and, perhaps more important, *content* with the natural ebbs and flows of your energy and output.

22.

Overcome procrastination.

One of the biggest barriers to productivity is procrastination. We set goals for ourselves, but when it comes down to actually progressing toward those goals, something often feels more inspiring in the moment. It could be doing the less daunting, more immediately rewarding task of answering emails, getting a dopamine hit from checking social media, or relaxing with a favorite TV show. So how can we learn to focus on and invest in our long-term goals, instead of getting caught up in the distractions that offer short-term rewards?

According to Dr. Katy Milkman, a Wharton professor who studies behavior change, the answer is commitment devices: self-imposed penalties designed to get us to stick to our goals. "It's like being your own manager," Dr. Milkman explained. "We're used to other people giving us deadlines with a penalty if we don't achieve them, and while it might feel odd to set them for ourselves, research shows it can be really useful."[1]

Commitment devices come in many forms. There are apps that financially penalize you if you don't reach your goals—for instance, if you don't walk a certain number of steps, stay off social media for a certain amount of time, or write a certain number of pages every day, a donation will be made to a cause you hate (which you select in advance). You can also use money as a commitment device by signing up for noncancelable services like a workout class (if your goal is exercising more) or a recurring grocery delivery filled with vegetables (if you want to eat more nutritious food). If you want to commit to actually using your vacation days (something that numerous studies show would benefit both productivity and physical health,[2] but that only about half of U.S. workers actually do[3]), pay for a nonrefundable hotel room.

There are also social commitment devices, like arranging to meet a friend for a walk or work session—the penalty of disappointing someone you care about is likely to help you honor your commitment.

If you have a task or a project that constantly seems to fall victim to procrastination, think about how you might employ commitment devices (they're even more powerful when combined with temptation bundling—see page 28—and creating bite-sized goals—see page 23) to help you accomplish your goals. Sometimes holding yourself accountable can be the kindest thing you can do for yourself.

23.

Artificially limit your time.

Productivity expert Chris Bailey has performed thousands of experiments on himself. When I had talked to him about productivity hacks, he shared one of my favorites, an exploration that proves that having more time does not always mean getting more done.

"For one month, I alternated between working ninety hours a week and twenty hours a week," he explained. "I realized that I accomplished only a little bit more during the ninety-hour weeks than I did during the twenty-hour weeks."

This can be attributed to a phenomenon called Parkinson's law, which states that our work tends to expand to fit how much time we have available for its completion. Because I, personally, am an excellent procrastinator, I've been able to discover the truth of this law in my own life. If I have a week to meet a deadline, somehow the work fills the entire week, but if I have a single day to meet a deadline, well—somehow the work gets finished that day.

Parkinson's law is thought to be true for several reasons. Our sense of how long a task will actually take is often wrong—we either overestimate it, or we *underestimate* it, and then fill the perceived "extra" time with nonessential tasks to procrastinate. We also use any resources available to us, but we can often make do with many fewer resources. Finally, it's a self-fulfilling prophecy: when we expect a task to take a certain amount of time, we adjust our schedule, pacing, and resources accordingly. Recently, this has been demonstrated on a grand scale in the UK, where they ran a pilot 32-hour workweek program with 2,900 workers at 61 companies. The results were astoundingly positive: 39 percent of employees were less stressed, and 71 percent had reduced levels of burnout at the end of the trial—all while organizations reported revenue increases of 35 percent on average when compared to similar periods from previous years.[1] Needlessly lengthening the time we designate to tasks is wasting our energy and increasing our levels of stress and burnout. Spending less time on the things we *have* to do frees up more precious time to do the things we *want* to do, the things that give meaning and purpose to our lives.

Today, try an experiment where you artificially limit your time. Give yourself fifteen minutes to tidy your house (this is quite literally the only way I can get myself to clean, and I'm always shocked at how much of a difference it makes!), or twenty minutes to go through all the emails in your inbox. Whatever amount of time you choose, make sure it's less than you would typically give yourself for the task you've selected. Artificially constraining my time has let me accomplish more than I ever thought possible (I'm doing it right now as I write this book!). I can't wait to see what it does for you.

24.

Direct your focus the
way you want to.

If you've ever had an undesirable thought stuck in your mind, University of Miami psychology professor and *Peak Mind* author Dr. Amishi Jha has two tricks for you. I spoke with her about how to direct our attention where we want it, which includes taking focus away from things we *don't* want to focus on.

To begin, it's important to understand the three systems of attention, which Dr. Jha calls flashlight, floodlight, and executive control. Our flashlight is what allows us to prioritize certain information over other information, zeroing in on it like a beam of light in the darkness. If you're focused on reading a book, or on someone's voice as they're talking, or on a particular thought, that's your flashlight system working.

The second system is the floodlight, which is a general alertness that makes you ready for anything that could happen. It's a broader type of attention that functions as almost the exact opposite of the flashlight.

Finally, the executive control system allows us to prioritize some information over other information based on our goals. "It ensures that the goals that we have and the actions that we engage in are aligned, and then corrects if there's a mismatch," said Dr. Jha.

If you're using your floodlight, it's harder to use your flashlight, and vice versa. "They're constantly battling each other," she said.

"If you think of the last time you were doing something really focused and somebody walked into the room and started talking to you, you probably wouldn't even hear them at first. The flashlight was activated, and executive control said, 'Yes, stay on this goal.'" The result of that is dialing down the functioning of the floodlight, because your attention is being utilized by the flashlight. It takes a moment to activate that other system.

When we're fixated on a sticky, unwelcome thought, our flashlight is essentially shining on that thought, and our job is to pull it away. When we're in those circumstances, Dr. Jha said, it can be helpful to either zoom out or zoom in.

"The zooming out is switching to the floodlight," said Dr. Jha. "The flashlight has its grip on you, but the second you realize you're stuck on a thought, you bring awareness to the situation, and you can use your executive control to get into what we call decentering mode. Zoom out. Visualize yourself as being in a traffic helicopter above yourself sitting there. Your job is to use third person and, in as granular a way as possible, report what's going on, but just exactly what you see, without making up any stories about it. 'She's feeling nervous. She's having that same anxious thought over and over again. She's feeling compression in her chest, she's feeling her jaw clench.'"

In that moment, because attention cannot be in two places at once, you're weakening the flashlight. "People will say their experience changes. 'Oh, her chest is now not as tight. She's noticing that there's less clenching in her jaw.' The anxious focused thoughts can dissipate, because we're pulling ourselves away instead of continuing to feed the direct experience. That's the zooming out."

You can also zoom in to have the same effect, hijacking the flashlight to turn on the floodlight system of attention. "Instead of zooming out and reporting on yourself from above, zoom in and check in on what's going on in your body," explained Dr. Jha. "Sit for a moment and ask what the most prominent physical sensation you have right now is. Really try to watch what's going on. Can you feel it in your chest? Your back? Do your feet feel tingly?"

By noticing your bodily sensations, you're weakening that grip on your flashlight. "You're not trying to yank the flashlight some-where else, which doesn't work," Dr. Jha said. "That's called the white bear phenomenon, where if I say, 'Don't think about a white bear. Don't think about a white bear,' what are you going to think about? A white bear." Instead, you're intentionally guiding your at-tention to a different system. "You're broadening your floodlight system. And because of that antagonistic relationship, when you're broad, it's hard to be focused."

The next time you find yourself facing a tenacious unwelcome thought, think about your systems of attention. How can you take advantage of this awareness to switch your focus? Can you zoom out or in to hijack your flashlight and activate your floodlight? I've found that even understanding the dichotomy between the two systems and the basic principle that they can't both work at once can be a game changer in my quest to regain control over my atten-tion. Throughout the day, I ask myself, *Am I in flashlight or flood-light mode? Is my flashlight where I want it to be?* and the practice has been, well—illuminating.

WANT TO DIVE DEEPER?

Listen to these episodes of The Liz Moody Podcast:

- "Productivity Secrets—How to Conquer Procrastination, Build a Better Morning Routine, and Get More Done in Less Time with Chris Bailey," episode 94

- "How to Hack Your Focus & Pay More Attention to the Things That Matter with Neuroscientist Dr. Amishi Jha," episode 106

Explore these resources from our expert guests:

- *The Productivity Project: Accomplishing More by Managing Your Time, Attention, and Energy* by Chris Bailey, www.chrisbailey.com

- *Peak Mind: Find Your Focus, Own Your Attention, Invest 12 Minutes a Day* by Dr. Amishi Jha, www.amishi.com

HOW TO INCREASE CREATIVITY

25.

Just start.

Josh Peck has accomplished a lot in the creative realm. He's starred in hit movies and television shows, written the bestselling memoir *Happy People Are Annoying,* hosted several podcasts, and created social media platforms that amuse and delight millions of people on a daily basis.

When I interviewed him, I asked him about his secret to success, and he quoted prolific YouTuber and entrepreneur Casey Neistat: "The right time is always right now."

"The good news is, there are no gatekeepers anymore," Peck said. "You don't need to live in a coastal city or have an agent or a manager to find success in the creative world. But there are also far fewer excuses. If you have a reasonable smartphone, you have enough video power to create content. So start. You have to start."

I've seen it happen over and over within my own social network—friends will get excited about a creative endeavor, and then spend the next six months getting in their own way. They need a better camera. They need to learn to edit better. They have to read a book or take a class on the subject. And while I'm a huge fan of educating yourself, I also think that a fundamental reason many people don't find success is that *they never begin.*

A lot of this is an unfortunate side effect of the fact that in today's world, we're constantly exposed to the people who have the great cameras, the great editing, the deep levels of knowledge—you can scroll briefly through a social media feed and see hundreds of people at the top of their game. When we normalize the expert end product, the gap between that and what we're capable of creating as beginners can feel insurmountable. When we compare our output to the output of people at peak levels of success, it's obvious that ours will fall short. But that doesn't remove the subconscious expectation, and it doesn't help us overcome the perfectionism that can stop us before we even begin. So we stall. We look at equipment online. We play around with a logo. We tell our friends about a plot twist in our novel. But we never write it.

The people you're comparing yourself to are where they are because one day, they got started. And on that day, their output was nowhere near what you're seeing now. In fact, they were probably pretty terrible at whatever they were doing. But there's no replacement for the learning that comes from doing, so little by little, they got better. They were able to assess public reaction and adjust. They were able to edit and tweak drafts. They were able to learn what certain light does at certain times of day, or which types of Photoshop tweaks were pleasing to their artistic eye. The difference between someone with a successful project and someone without one is often—not always, but often—simply that one day, the successful person began.

"When I started my YouTube channel, it was dismal for a year," shared Peck. "But that year was an R-and-D time for me to figure out what I was doing that didn't work. And the main thing that didn't work was that I wasn't being truthful to who I was. We all have that special something. My acting teacher always says, 'Embrace your sparkle.' It's that willingness to be honest with who you are and what you want to convey."

To find your sparkle, you might need to imitate other people for a while. Joan Didion famously typed out Ernest Hemingway's novels to get a sense for the flow and rhythm of a well-written sentence. But through writing more, through practice, she found her own voice—and that voice eventually reached millions.

Another barrier to creative production is waiting for that spark of inspiration. "Somebody asked me how I found inspiration to write," said Tara Schuster, bestselling author of *Buy Yourself the*

*F*cking Lilies* and *Glow in the F*cking Dark*. "If I needed to be inspired to write, I would never write, because the number of times I've been inspired has been zero. It's overwhelming if you have to be inspired to write. It's just not sustainable."

Instead of focusing on that elusive creative drive, Schuster focuses on the *practice* of her work. "Writing is a habit. It's not some magical, mysterious thing," she said. By eliminating the enticing enigma of creative work, Schuster is also able to eliminate expectations that might keep her from being able to do that work. "Before I write, I visualize that I've put a cardboard box on my desk. In the cardboard box, I put the word 'good,' and then I put the word 'interesting.' Then I close the box, I tape it up, and I throw it off my desk, because it's not my job to make this good or interesting," she said. "My only task is to show up, write, and do the best that I can in that moment. The rest is for other people to decide."

What story do you want to tell? What kind of art or business do you want to create? Whatever it is, pick a time this week and get started. Set the bar low—write fifty words, google "how to make a business plan"—but get started. And then do it the next day, and the next. I've seen novels written in stolen half hours before the kids wake up, and products brought to life in one-hour sessions scheduled during lunchtime. You have everything you need, I promise. What you produce might not be good, but I can tell you this—it will get better. You'll learn by doing, and someday, you'll look back and be so grateful to the person you are this week, who finally put pen to paper or clicked open their computer. Now is the time to begin.

26.

Gesture and fidget more.

Acclaimed science writer and *The Extended Mind* author Annie Murphy Paul thinks most of us are missing out on tapping into the true power of our minds. Her research focuses on moving beyond brain-based thinking and into the many other ways our outside-the-brain resources can literally help us get smarter.

As it turns out, gesturing is one of the ways our interaction with our bodies actually changes how we think. "Linguists think that gesture was probably our first language, before we even were able as a species to use spoken language to communicate, and we still communicate through gestures," Paul said.

According to Paul, though, gesturing isn't just about communicating with other people—it actually assists and enhances our own thinking as well. "There are amazing experiments that show that our gestures are a few milliseconds ahead of our verbal expressions and even our conscious thoughts in terms of what we're about to say," she explained. "We can actually read information off of our own gestures that will help us find the right words or locate the right concepts."

Gesturing can also increase our capacity for memory recall. Numerous studies have found that gesturing when trying to recall a word or memory can bring something from that tip-of-the-tongue state to the more accessible part of the brain,[1] and recently, research has shown that when people gesture while they're *encoding* a memory, that memory is later more easily recalled.[2] Speakers remember their speeches better if there are actions associated with the words; actors who use gesturing better recall their scripts; children who gesture while learning are more likely to retain what they learned than children who stay still.

To cheat the bodily process that's already happening, you can allow and encourage gesturing, especially when you're trying to enhance your thinking. "The more we gesture, the deeper our understanding of a concept will be. As workers, thinkers, and creators, we want to allow ourselves to gesture as much as possible," shared Paul.

On the flip side, a lot of our mental resources are used up when we try to inhibit our urge to move (and this can be even more true for neurodiverse people). "We actually have to devote mental bandwidth just to keeping ourselves still," Paul said, "whereas fidgeting is actually a very finely modulated way of adjusting our own arousal level. It might keep us awake during a boring meeting, or if we're kind of playing with some kind of object on our desk, that might sort of put us in a more creative frame of mind. I would love to see us give ourselves more permission to fidget, to doodle, to gesture, and not feel like those things are somehow anti-intellectual. They're actually enhancing our thinking."

As a very small personal example, when I used to do my podcast intro and outro recordings, I'd feel silly for the gestures that my body naturally felt compelled to make. I remember once even sitting on my hands—I'd so internalized that gestures were a signal you sent *to* other people, and no one else was in the room with me, after all. Who was I trying to communicate with?

Since my interview with Paul, though, I've allowed myself to gesture wildly because, as she explained, it's really a signal I'm sending to myself. And I've found that my thoughts flow more freely when my hands are waving around like I'm conducting an orchestra. Sentences come easier; words feel more graspable. Explore incorporating gestures when you talk. If you're trying to memorize something, incorporate a gesture that goes with the words that you're committing to memory. When you're trying to recall something, move your hands and arms and see if it helps spark the memory. Also, try to become aware of when you're *limiting* your gestures, whether it's to adhere to some social norm or for any other reason—because, as Paul points out, you're not simply limiting your movement, but the power of your mind as well.

27.

Do nothing (with intention).

Looking to supercharge your creativity? According to Dr. Tara Swart Bieber, a neuroscientist who teaches at MIT Sloan and King's College London and the author of *The Source*, doing absolutely nothing—with the right intention—is one of the most powerful ways to hack our neurobiology.

"The neuroscience shows that if you're getting distracted into daydreaming when you're trying to focus, that's not good," she explained. "But if you sit and you *allow* your mind to wander, you move it from the control network to the default network, which aligns with creative thinking." In fact, according to Dr. Swart Bieber, it activates a completely different hormone and neurotransmitter profile. "Your brain knows the difference between when you've done something on purpose or not," she says.

When we do nothing, Dr. Swart Bieber says, we're activating an entire system of our brain that in our daily lives is often turned on far less than the control network. "It's the part of your brain that lets you think flexibly, that lets you see patterns that aren't necessarily obvious to everyone and come up with creative ideas," she said.

A variation of this idea also came up in my interview with acclaimed science writer Annie Murphy Paul. "There's really compelling research on what psychologists call incubation,[1] which is the fact that even when we're not consciously thinking about a problem, our nonconscious mind will continue to puzzle on it,"

Paul explained. "But you're not giving your nonconscious mind a chance to noodle on a problem if you're maintaining this really rigid focus. This is exactly why most people will tell you that they get good ideas in the shower or when they're taking a walk or taking a bike ride—because that's when the default network in the brain takes over, and we get these sort of more free-flowing associative thoughts. That's where a lot of our best ideas are going to come from."

I've found that doing nothing is most useful in two scenarios: First, when I'm feeling stuck on a problem I'm trying to solve. Paul pointed out that while often we want to sit at our computer and power through until we come to a solution, our brains will serve us best if we do the exact opposite, stepping away and letting the problem incubate. This is easier said than done—literally the only thing that gets my overly productivity-focused self up and out of my chair is telling myself over and over that *the science supports stepping away*, that stepping away is what will solve the problem, not staring at my flashing cursor and retyping sentences for the next hour.

The second is embracing the small moments of nothing that naturally pop up in my life—taking a shower, going for a walk, waiting for my tea water to boil, or sitting at a red light. These are moments I'd normally try to grab my phone, pick up a book, do *something*, anything, just to—to be completely frank—avoid the squirmy unease of being alone with my own brain. After interviewing Dr. Swart Bieber, though, I relish the opportunity to do nothing, to intentionally let my brain bounce from one place to another. I sometimes picture my neurons flicking on lights in dusty, cobweb-filled folds of my brain tissue, an image that helped me power through the palpable discomfort the exercise caused, especially at the beginning. But it's gotten easier. Now I find myself looking forward to these daily doses of nothing, which feel sometimes even more powerful than all the *somethings* I speckle my life with.

Take a break not only because you deserve it (you always deserve it), but because it will get you closer to your overall goals and solutions. I promise.

28.

Run into an "aha!" moment.

While doing nothing can be extremely beneficial for getting the creative wheels turning (see page 93), if you're the type of person who feels antsy at the prospect of inaction, research has your back there: it turns out science supports engaging in a specific type of exercise to stoke creativity as well.

"When people run at a very fast pace for a sustained amount of time, the brain is so consumed with the demands of that kind of high-intensity exercise that the prefrontal cortex, which is the part of the brain that judges, criticizes, plans, and does those sort of higher-level mental activities, dials down its activity, because there's so much going on in terms of just controlling the body and its movements," explained acclaimed science writer Annie Murphy Paul. "That state of prefrontal cortex occupation also takes place in dream states or when you're having a drug trip. It's when ideas and associations can collide and combine in really creative ways."

If you need creative inspiration, one way to get there is to physically exhaust your body to a point where you're not thinking in a cerebral, judgmental way. You can also maximize this process by being very explicit about the question you pose to yourself before the workout. "Set the problem or challenge to yourself in very clear and explicit terms. 'How can I make this introduction flow into the first chapter?' 'How can I frame this presentation in a really compelling way?'" Paul shared.

If you have a problem you can't solve, you can try a couple of different approaches: doing less (see page 71), or disengaging your prefrontal cortex by doing a high-intensity workout. Go for a fast run. Put on a loud song and dance until you're out of breath. Physically occupy your body, and see what solutions pop up.

WANT TO DIVE DEEPER?

Listen to this episode of The Liz Moody Podcast:

- "How to Literally Become Smarter with Annie Murphy Paul," episode 149

Explore these resources from our expert guests:

- *The Extended Mind: The Power of Thinking Outside the Brain* by Annie Murphy Paul, @anniemurphypaul on Twitter

HOW TO
BE MORE
SUCCESSFUL

29.

Get in motion.

In the late 1600s, mathematician Isaac Newton established the first law of thermodynamics, asserting that an object at rest stays at rest, and an object in motion stays in motion. This law forever changed the way scientists understood the idea of energy transfer. Several hundred years later, it also helped me get my butt off the couch.

I was procrastinating one day, phone in hand, my body melting into the cushions. I had work to do; I *knew* I had work to do; the voice in my head kept telling me I had work to do, among other less kind sentiments my inner critic has been known to suggest. But I couldn't stop scrolling. And from a Newtonian perspective, it made sense: I was at rest. Inertia meant that the easiest path forward was to stay at rest.

And then I realized: the key was to change my state in the simplest possible way. Objects in motion *stay* in motion, so I needed to get into *any* motion. Trying to actually accomplish my task for work was too large of a state change, but if I could do something easier to get in motion, I could capitalize on that motion to ultimately execute the thing I was supposed to do from the start. Instead of pushing myself to get up and start working, I set the bar much lower—I made a cup of tea. Once I was up, my limbs having regained their solid state, it was indeed much easier to make my next move, to my computer. I stayed in motion until my work was complete.

The next time you're procrastinating, take the smallest, least intimidating possible step toward motion. Make a cup of tea. Do five jumping jacks. Go brush your teeth. Put in a load of laundry. Send a single email. I keep a note of possible motions on my phone so that when I'm stuck in a procrastination cycle, I don't even have to make the effort of thinking of something to do—I can just pick something off the list.

Once you're in motion, inertia will propel you forward. Every time I use this trick, I'm shocked at how well it works. But then again, I was never that good at physics.

30.

Identify your
financial dreams.

One of the many things I love about Ramit Sethi is that he's a financial expert who encourages people to think about how to *spend* their money as much as how to save it. After your basic needs are met, the point of having money, after all, is to use it to create *your* unique, satisfying Rich Life. "Most of us have gone thirty, forty years, never actually deciding what do we want to do with our money," he said when I interviewed him on the podcast. "What is our Rich Life?"

It's a startling thought: many of us are so focused on the saving side of the equation (which is important, to be sure—Sethi and other financial experts recommend automating as much of that process as possible; see page 61) that we never stop to think about *why* we want to accumulate wealth in the first place. If we spend the majority of our waking hours trying to acquire something we're not intentional about spending, we're wasting, at least in part, those waking hours. It's a sobering thought, but don't worry: Sethi has spent his life developing an antidote.

One of the biggest problems is that from a spending perspective, many of us don't know what will actually make us happy. For the whole of our lives, we've been subject to societal messaging about wanting the great house and the nice car and the dream wedding and the fun vacations. How do we evaluate whether a sabbatical, a weekly professional home cleaning, or a beautiful, chic wardrobe is our Rich Life? How do we know what luxuries will truly make us happier? I asked Sethi, and he suggested asking ourselves two questions to figure out what constitutes our personal Rich Life.

Question number one: What do you love to spend money on? "The most common answers are eating out, travel, and then health and wellness, in that order," shared Sethi. "Personally, I love spending money on convenience." Note that Sethi's answer isn't the most common one, and that's *okay*. A key element of a Rich Life is that it's *yours*. Cutting through the noise of what your parents, your friends, advertisements, and social media are telling you constitutes a good life is a critical part of the exercise. Figuring out the difference between what you're *told* you should love spending money on versus what you *actually* love spending money on is the key to living *your* Rich Life—otherwise, you're simply spending years of your life working to fill other people's pockets and fulfill other people's dreams. The day I realized I didn't care about status cars was incredibly freeing, as was the day I first questioned whether home ownership was even a goal of mine (Sethi himself has fairly radical thoughts about home ownership—namely, that it is by no means a necessary or even recommended path to wealth for many people). Figuring out what you *don't* care about spending money on frees you up to use your money to create your Rich Life. "You probably don't care equivalently about a wedding as a scarf," Sethi explained. "One of them is more meaningful to you— I don't know which. But when you start with what you love, suddenly, it becomes easier to cut back on things that you don't care about."

Still stuck on determining what, outside all the external noise, you *truly* love? That's where question two comes in: What would it look like if you could quadruple your spending on that thing? How would it feel? This exercise helps separate what we might enjoy spending a bit more money on ("It'd be *nice* to have a few more pairs of shoes") from the things that truly light us up ("If I could go to the theater every week, it would transform my life!"). And those things that truly light you up? Those need to be the focus of your

Rich Life. And after your basic needs are taken care of, *those* are the things you should be spending your money on.

Ask yourself: What is your ultimate goal or purpose in wanting to earn money? What do you love to spend money on? What would your life look like if you could spend even more money on the thing you value most? Our financial health touches almost every part of our ability to be truly *well*, yet it's largely ignored in favor of thinking about supplements, meditation, or the new fitness craze. Yes, meditation and movement relieve stress (see pages 251 and 252 for more on that!), but no amount of sitting or running will bring you to a true baseline if you have underlying fiscal anxiety or if you're in essence wasting hours of work by blowing your earnings on things other people want for you.

What is your Rich Life? Why are you making money? How can you use your money to move in the direction of your dreams? What are some things other people might value that truly don't matter to you? Can you eliminate or reduce your spending on them?

Figure out what you value, and, as much as humanly possible, spend your money on that and only that. We all deserve a Rich Life. Take a second to figure out yours, and move relentlessly toward it.

31.

Amp up your charisma.

While charisma might feel indefinable and enigmatic, researchers have, in fact, pinpointed its exact components—and the good news is, they're accessible to all of us. You don't need to be an extrovert to be charismatic. You don't need to fit a societal definition of beauty. You just need to embody two key traits.

Vanessa Van Edwards, the bestselling author of *Captivate* and *Cues*, shared that the two traits that very charismatic people signal to others, whether consciously or not, are warmth (characterized by words like "likability," "friendliness," "approachability," "collaborativeness") and competence (characterized by words like "power," "capability," "memorability," "efficiency"). "The key here is to evidence a balance of both," explained Van Edwards. "If you have an imbalance—too much warmth without enough competence, or too much competence without enough warmth—you're not seen as charismatic. That sweet spot of being both *likable* and *powerful* is the definition of high charisma."

While people exhibit these traits in varying amounts naturally (that's why we're hardwired to respond positively to them!), there are ways to hack the system and amp up what Van Edwards calls your cues, which can signal your warmth or your competence. "A head tilt is a universal sign of warmth," she explained. "It's what humans do across cultures, genders, and races when they're trying to listen better—we tilt our head and we expose our ear, because that's literally our physically best listening position." Van Edwards has identified other nonverbal warmth cues—a wave with a visible palm, a nod hello, a smile—and verbal ones as well, like vocalizations. "Saying things like 'hmm' and 'oh' are super high in warmth. They make us feel heard and understood. They're very similar to the sounds our mothers made to soothe us to sleep. Use them when someone is speaking to be heard without being loud—this is great for introverts as well. They're super encouraging, and charismatic people are great at them."

And then there are competence cues. One of the most interesting competence cues that Van Edwards shared was a concept called maximizing, which means literally maximizing the space between your earlobe and your shoulder. According to her, this physical shift—of taking up more space in moments of pride or confidence—is a consistent behavior in cultures and societies across the world in people viewed as competent. "Specifically, they tend to keep their head angled up, their shoulders down, their body relaxed and open wide. They have no barriers between themselves and others," she said. "In defeat, losing athletes do the opposite. They typically tuck their chin to their chest. They roll their shoulders in and down. When we're in defeat, we want to protect our jugular, our vital organs. We cross our arms over our body and pin our arms tightly to our torso. You want to make sure that the space between your ear and your shoulder is maximized. That is the single fastest way to show someone you're open. You're not protected, you're confident, you're relaxed."

Start by taking an intuitive survey of where you fall on the warmth/competence spectrum. Do you naturally tend to be a little higher in warmth, or competence? Try to add cues of the trait you feel you tend toward *less*. "Highly charismatic people dial up their warmth when they need it and dial up their competence when they need it," Van Edwards explained. Becoming aware of your warmth and competence and working to deploy both traits as needed will forever change how you're perceived and received in the world.

32.

Start an advice club.

Receiving advice can obviously be beneficial, but it turns out there are also benefits to offering someone else a few words of wisdom.

"When we coach and mentor others who have similar goals, it also helps us," shared behavior change expert Dr. Katy Milkman. "When we're advising others, someone's looking up to us, and that makes us feel like we have something to offer, boosts our confidence, and forces us to introspect about what could be an effective tool, which helps dredge up insights that we wouldn't have thought of otherwise. If you're trying to help someone else, you're going to think harder and more deeply, and make sure that you have something to say."

Sharing advice will build your confidence and solidify your knowledge of that subject matter. On top of this, once you've given that advice to someone else, you're going to feel hypocritical if you don't follow it yourself, which, again, helps you improve your own performance. In fact, research shows that people are overwhelmingly more motivated by giving advice than receiving it.

There are many compelling ways to apply this research in everyday life: you can explain to a friend a concept that you're trying to nail down yourself, or take on a mentorship position in your career (you can also simply pretend you're advising a best friend). Dr. Milkman, though, created an ingenious way to simultaneously experience the benefits of giving *and* receiving advice, all while adding the myriad researched benefits of forming community: she created an Advice Club. The club is composed of a group of female professionals at comparable career stages at different universities. They have similar goals and work in similar environments, and regularly reach out to each other when facing challenges. The benefits have far exceeded Dr. Milkman's expectations.

"We knew it would build a community," she said. "We knew we'd get brilliant insights that would help us make better choices. But an aspect that I didn't appreciate going in was that when I'm asked for advice, it helps me think more carefully and clearly about how to handle a given situation. We often have blinders on when it's our own challenge. We can get emotional about it and lose perspective. But when it's someone else's challenge, I think much more clearly, and that builds my confidence that I can do this for myself, too."

When you're forming your Advice Club, make sure you choose people you trust, and that the club's collective goal is to reinforce positive beliefs rather than negative ones. "You may want to look for a group who has faced similar challenges," said Dr. Milkman. "My Advice Club is a group of female professionals, and that's very deliberate, because I think there's different barriers we face, and we can build each other up and give advice that's relevant to members of our identity group."

As someone who's long lamented my lack of ability to find a mentor, the concept of an Advice Club felt like a breath of fresh air. I could be mentored by a group of people all at once, and at the same time, I could experience the real emotional and intellectual results of sharing my wisdom with other people. I started an Advice Club with other female podcast hosts who have found success in a male-dominated space. On our text chain, we share everything from advertising insights to quandaries about types of content. We cheer on each other's wins and champion each other through losses. We gain perspective and guidance not only from each other, but from considering and reconsidering situations ourselves.

Is there an area of your life that would benefit from an Advice Club? Reach out to someone you'd be interested in kicking it off with (if you're nervous, just assume people like you). Explore the myriad ways that receiving *and* giving advice can benefit your life.

33.

Identify your unique gifts.

This concept came out of an interview I did with business and career coach Amina AlTai, and I immediately thought it was genius, both because it gave me the opportunity to ask people for compliments, and because it's a really helpful way to gain a new perspective on our lives.

"We have our gifts, which are the areas where we are just off-the-charts amazing," AlTai explained. "Our gifts are innate for us. We don't have to push or force ourselves to be amazing at them. It's just what comes through us naturally."

According to AlTai, we want to operate in those exceptional zones as much as possible. "When we stand in that area, versus what we're simply good at, what we contribute is so expansive. Conversely, when we push or force to make ourselves good at things we're fundamentally not designed for, we use so much energy and mindshare that it can lead to or exacerbate burnout."

If you're unsure what your gifts actually are, fear not—AlTai has specific questions that you can ask yourself to begin your journey:

- When do you find yourself in the state of flow? What are you doing or sharing?
- When you walk into a room, what do you bring in that wasn't there before?

- When you're on a project, what are you bringing that wasn't there before?
- What are the things that people reflect to you as your most exceptional abilities?

If you want to take it to the next level, you can text a few people you feel truly know you and ask them what they think your unique gifts are. AlTai underscored the importance of reaching out to people in your life who see you fully and want the best for you, and avoiding people who might have a tendency to project. It's scary—and I know that because I actually tried this exercise. I texted people from different parts of my life—my sister, my best friend from my previous job, an old roommate from college, and a former boss I was still in touch with—to get as wide a cross-section of opinions as possible. It might feel awkward (and if it does, just tell them it's for an exercise you're doing!), but you'll likely be surprised by how responsive and receptive people are—and how their insights both overlap and differ. Seeing them answer things about being a good question asker, a risk taker, and an executor not only felt amazing, but helped inform choices that I was making at the time. It also teased out parts that I rarely give myself credit for—almost everyone said I was a hard worker, while I often view myself as lazy, and hearing them speak to my kindness and interest in helping others made my life feel full of meaning and purpose (I have their full responses on my Instagram Reels, @lizmoody, if you'd like to see).

AlTai also suggested keeping a folder on your phone or computer where you can keep emails that highlight positive feedback you've received. I personally have a folder in my photos on my iPhone, and when people send me complimentary DMs or write touching podcast reviews, I screenshot them and put the screenshots in this folder. When I find myself questioning my own gifts, or wondering what my purpose is in the world, I open the folder and flip through the screenshots. It's been affirming, reading the words of people who've praised my communication skills or shared the life impact of listening to my podcast, but also directionally clarifying when I'm at decision points in my career. It's a win-win; it feels good, and, as AlTai said, "There's probably breadcrumbs in there for where you are off-the-charts genius."

Look—we can't all operate in our zone of genius 100 percent of the time. We have bills to pay, economic systems to deal with, family circumstances that limit us. But it's all about the ratio. "When it comes to joy and gifts, I have a sixty-forty rule," AlTai said. "If sixty percent of the time you feel like you're on the court with your gifts and you're feeling a sense of joy, that's a really wonderful thing. We all have aspects of our roles that we find challenging or that don't always feel amazing. It's a privilege to operate in our zone of genius all day every day, but if we're taking one step towards it each day, we're doing great."

And it's *recognizing* that you have your own particular genius parts, figuring out what they are, and moving toward them as much as possible that will move you *away* from burnout, directionlessness, and feeling a lack of purpose.

34.

Overcome impostor syndrome.

I want to raise my hand right now and say: "I struggle with impostor syndrome." There have been days I've sat down to write this very book or host the podcast it's based on and thought: *Why me? Surely there's someone else more qualified or talented who people should be spending their precious time with.*

You know who else has their hands raised? *Almost every single world-class expert and top performer I've ever talked to.* Bestselling authors. Scientists who helmed studies that have changed the way we think. CEOs. Models. Professional athletes.

The first step to overcoming impostor syndrome is realizing that the vast majority of people have it. That person you think is more qualified to take your place, who you're sure would be so much better at performing than you? They probably have impostor syndrome too. Some studies show that as many as 82 percent of us struggle with this often unconscious belief that deep down we're not as intelligent, capable, competent, qualified, or talented as other people think we are.[1]

"It's counterintuitive, because we can see the degree on the wall," said Valerie Young, who authored *The Secret Thoughts of Successful Women* and cofounded the Impostor Syndrome Institute. "We can see concrete evidence of our abilities, and yet we chalk them up to outside factors—things like luck, timing, computer error—and we're left with this fear of being found out."

The good news is, there are pragmatic steps you can take to free yourself from the binds of impostor syndrome. First up: recognizing our bias for negative information.

"With impostor syndrome, we have this trick scale where only the negative evidence counts. You give a talk, and ninety-nine people say it was great, but one person says it was the worst talk they've ever been to, and you believe that one person. We think everyone else was just being nice," said Young.

To combat that sense, Young suggested zooming out to gain a sense of perspective. "You don't like every book. You don't like every film. We don't like everything. Why should everybody like us?" she shared. "It's about making a conscious decision: 'I'm going to focus on the ninety-nine percent of people for whom I am their cup of tea.' And those other people will be well-served to go somewhere else, which is a better fit for them."

It's a simple thought but a radical one: not everyone is going to like me, *and that is okay.* If you focus on the people for whom your message is a good fit rather than chasing down the people for whom it never will be, you'll be spending your time far more efficiently and saving large amounts of mental energy (which will, interestingly, actually free up the capacity for you to perform better at your task of choice).

Another way to get a reality check is to ask yourself, *And then what?*

"I know people who've had money and had time and they still couldn't get out of their own way to start a business or take a risk," Young said. "They're overwhelmed by this fear of 'Can I do it? What will people think? Will I fail? Am I smart enough? Do I know enough?'"

Let's say you do fail. And then what? Let's say the speech goes terribly. And then what? Chances are, the results will be far *less* catastrophic than they are in your head, and on the flip side, you'll be far *more* resilient and better equipped to deal with the situation. Young also recommends actively seeking out criticism, asking your boss or colleagues or friends for ways you can improve. That way, you'll begin to reframe it not as something that points out why you *can't* do something, but rather as helpful information that enables you to do something *better*.

You can also watch out for moments where you undermine your own qualifications. Do any of these sound familiar?

"I can't believe I got them to pay me this much."

"My colleague is way more qualified to run that meeting."

"I'm not *really* a podcast host/author/engineer/expert in this subject."

"It was just luck."

"Anyone could have done it."

Whether you're saying it out loud to others or just to yourself, *your brain is hearing you*, and it's taking in that message. You're reinforcing the belief system over and over, building those neural connections, solidifying those patterns of thought, and making the statement feel more and more true.

Instead, try focusing on the facts at hand: They *did* pay you this much. You *are* running the meeting. You *host* a podcast; while perhaps anyone could have done it, you were the one that actually *did*. Keep a running list of wins you've had—proof points of your success—on your phone or computer and consult it in moments of self-doubt. If someone compliments you, you don't need to deflect—simply say thank you. Say, "I'm proud of what I've accomplished." We often think that confidence is something that precedes action, when in truth, confidence comes from *taking action—regardless of how we feel when we take it*.

"We have this sense that when we're confident, we'll do all of these things we desire," said therapist Vanessa Marin. "But when we take some sort of action, that's actually what builds confidence. We take a step, even if it's a teeny-tiny little step, and we realize that we did it. We were courageous and tried something different. We *survived*. That's what builds confidence."

Which brings me to the last step for overcoming impostor syndrome: do the thing anyway. If the majority of the world would feel unqualified in your same situation, nothing is gained by

swapping one of them in for you. The people who are most suc-
cessful aren't the people who are free from impostor syndrome;
they're the people who don't let impostor syndrome hold them
back. By thanking your brain for the input but still going after
your dreams, little by little, you're *demonstrating* to your mind
that you are competent and capable. You're overcoming your be-
liefs with actions until the beliefs no longer have any proof to fall
back on. "I want to say you're not qualified, but look at all the
meetings you've led before," your brain will muse. "Look at the
stages you've dominated. Look at the perspectives you've shifted
by sharing your own utterly unique take on the world."

Your impostor syndrome isn't a deficit. It's a fact of life, and
learning to push forward *regardless* is how you'll begin to take
your power back.

35.

Use neuroscience to bring your dreams to life.

As someone who falls more easily toward skepticism than belief, I've been dismissive of vision boards for years. Then I talked to famed neuroscientist and medical doctor Dr. Tara Swart Bieber, and she explained the science behind the practice to me.

"We're bombarded with so much information all the time," said Dr. Swart Bieber. "The brain has become very good at filtering out information that isn't relevant to our survival, and it's very much focused on that survival. It's not really thinking, 'What can I do to thrive and become successful and take lots of risks?'"

Your brain can *help* you create your best life, but to encourage that behavior, you have to intentionally prime it. By creating a vision board, Dr. Swart Bieber explained, you're telling your brain that it's safe, that it can move its attention from keeping you alive to focusing on the things that you want to thrive, a process called selective filtering. "It's giving your brain the message that you have enough food to survive, you have a safe place to sleep, and that the things you would like more than those basic things you already have to survive are x, y, and z," said Dr. Swart Bieber. "Then something called selective attention makes it so that you are more likely to notice the things that will lead you to whatever your goals for manifestation are." This is a process you've already experienced if you've ever become aware of a word and then suddenly seen that word everywhere, or gone car shopping and then noticed the models you were eyeing all over the streets. The cars were always there; what changed is the way you directed your focus.

Next, you need to add "value tagging," or consciously identifying what's important in your life so your brain can assign importance accordingly. Making what Dr. Swart Bieber calls an "action board," a step beyond a vision board, combines selective filtering, selective attention, and value tagging into one simple practice.

Why an action board? "For too long, there has been this idea that you can sit at home and create a fantasy ideal life and just do nothing and wait for it to come true. Based on neuroscience, I'm not a proponent of that belief," Dr. Swart Bieber explained. "It's actually better for your brain, your sense of agency, and your belief in your ability if you can show yourself what *you* did to make those results happen." Connecting your visions to specific actions that you'll take to achieve them makes them far more likely to happen (WOOP goals can be helpful for this; see page 25).

If you're not sure what you want on your action board—if you're not sure what direction you want your life to go—Dr. Swart Bieber says to represent a feeling instead of concrete items. Yes, putting a dollar amount you're going for is great; putting a country you want to travel to is amazing. If you have concrete goals, represent them as specifically as possible. But you can also look for images or words that you're drawn to without knowing why.

You can make your board online, or using physical cutouts from magazines and foam board—the key is just creating something that you see regularly so your brain can benefit from the three aforementioned cognitive processes that the visual triggers. Dr. Swart Bieber recommends creating a new action board once a year.

After her years of neuroplasticity research, she cited action boards as the biggest change maker in her arsenal. Pick a time (maybe a fresh start moment; see page 20) and make an action board. Harness the power of neuroscience to take a step toward the life of your dreams.

36.

Never be the one to
say no to yourself.

Here's a secret: I probably didn't deserve my first book deal. When I got it, I'd been developing recipes seriously for only six months or so, and I'd just recently switched my general journalism to a stronger wellness focus (a result of that bout of extreme agoraphobia I detailed in the introduction, which, frankly, I was still on the tail end of even as I pitched the book).

But when I had the idea for a cookbook of healthy ice pop recipes, I didn't ask myself, *Why would they let you write that?* Instead, I googled, "what does a cookbook proposal look like?" I found a few examples online and spent the next few weeks testing and photographing different recipes. I'd regularly have panic attacks when I left the house—and the house in question was my in-laws', where my husband and I were living while he got his post-grad school start-up off the ground and I wrote freelance and tried to recover my mental health. But still, I had a dream. I googled "how to find an agent" and began sending my proposal around. (You'll be shocked at how much highly specific, step-by-step advice is available on the internet. If you have no idea where to begin, start broad—"how do I publish a book?"—and then zero in on the details as you learn what those details are—"what makes a good query letter?")

Within two weeks, I had representation. Within a month, I was in New York, wearing the exact same outfit day after day as my agent and I traipsed around the city, meeting with editors at the biggest publishing houses in the world. I still remember the black silk pants, white silk shirt, and gold necklace, and I still remember apologetically telling my agent I couldn't afford more than one "professional author" costume. "I won't tell if you won't," she said.

Almost everyone we met with bid on the book, and we sold it at auction to a division of Penguin Random House. The advance from the book and some early success in Zack's start-up allowed us to move out of his parents' house and into a street-side walk-up in Williamsburg, Brooklyn, where every morning at 5 a.m., the same man would wake us up with his rendition of Whitney Houston songs as he made his way to work. That book, *Glow Pops*, was a key contributor to me landing my dream job at a wellness media site, where I worked my way up to food director. I ran the food section, and suddenly I had access to both the world's best chefs and the world's best doctors and could accumulate the cooking and health knowledge that began to make me feel less like an impostor in the food space. I landed a second book deal, for *Healthier Together*, a project larger in both advance and scope.

With all the connections I'd built and skills I'd honed, I launched *The Liz Moody Podcast*, and eventually left the traditional media world to act as the editor in chief of my own magazine, in the form of my social media content and podcast. Now I host one of the top personal growth podcasts in the world, I'm writing my third book (and the one that feels far and away the most "me"), I run a conversation card company with my husband, and I have millions of amazing community members with whom I get to explore all my biggest passions and curiosities. And it all happened because I didn't say no to myself.

"Never be the one to say no to yourself" has been a motto that's governed my life, and I attribute much of my success to it. It's not a free ticket to achieving your wildest dreams—there are still opportunities you're simply not qualified for or the right fit for, not to mention very real systemic inequities to contend with. Rather, it's an assurance that *you* won't be the one standing in your own way.

Every agent I reached out to could have said no to me. Even if I got an agent, every publishing house could've said, "No one wants to buy a book about ice pops," or "Thanks, but we'd rather have a *real* chef write this." But they didn't. And the *reason* I get to know that they didn't is because I didn't say no to myself.

Since sharing my motto in a viral social media post, I've gotten to hear thousands of stories from people who received raises tens of thousands of dollars higher than they could've hoped for; who asked the person of their dreams on a date and are now married; who wrote a heartfelt note to a house owner and were picked to be the buyer over people with better offers. I've heard from other people who've gotten book deals and recording contracts and hotel upgrades and dream jobs. And I've heard from people who heard no. I've heard thousands of nos in my own life—from guests I've pitched for my podcast and people I've asked out on friend dates, from my bosses when I still worked for an outside organization. And guess what? *It still feels better.*

Because here's the thing: while never being the one to say no to yourself gives you access to the life of your dreams, it also gives you access to a different relationship with yourself. Instead of being the one beating yourself down, telling yourself you don't deserve things, you become your own biggest cheerleader. You start to see yourself as a person who is worthy of living the life of your dreams, and if other people don't recognize that, well—that's their problem. There will be yeses for you elsewhere. And every day, at every moment, you're giving yourself the biggest yes of them all.

Look around your life and find one way you're saying no to yourself. Maybe it's a new friendship you've been holding back on cultivating for fear of rejection. Maybe it's a career change. Maybe it's a new structure of household labor with your partner. Maybe it's writing a book, or asking out that person you've been eyeing at the gym. Whatever it is, do the research to set yourself up for success as much as you can, and then go for it. Seek out the no. And don't be surprised when it's actually a yes.

WANT TO DIVE DEEPER?

Listen to these episodes of The Liz Moody Podcast:

- "Science Hacks to Make ANYONE More Charismatic at Work, at Parties, on Dates, and in Relationships with Vanessa Van Edwards," episode 111
- "Ramit Sethi Answers YOUR Money Questions," episode 119
- "How to Be Happier at Work: Burn Out, Knowing When You Need to Make a Big Change, Beating the Sunday Scaries & More with Amina AlTai," episode 123
- "How to Overcome Impostor Syndrome and Start Living Your Best Life with Dr. Valerie Young," episode 117

Explore these resources from our expert guests:

- *Cues: Master the Secret Language of Charismatic Communication* by Vanessa Van Edwards, ScienceofPeople.com
- *I Will Teach You to Be Rich: No Guilt. No Excuses. No BS. Just a 6-Week Program That Works*, 2nd edition, by Ramit Sethi, IWillTeachYouToBeRich.com
- Amina AlTai, www.aminaaltai.com
- *The Secret Thoughts of Successful Women: Why Capable People Suffer from the Impostor Syndrome and How to Thrive in Spite of It* by Dr. Valerie Young, www.impostorsyndrome.com

HOW TO
LOVE YOURSELF

37.

Keep a promise to yourself.

There's a lot of talk in the wellness world about loving yourself, and very little pragmatic instruction on how to actually do it. Jamie Varon, author of *Radically Content*, wants to change that—and her approach is vastly different than the action-free platitudes that saturate the self-help space.

"You don't want to start with self-love," she shared. "You want to start with self-trust, because if you're saying you love yourself, but you don't trust yourself, you're essentially lying to yourself. You're saying: 'I love you, but I don't act lovingly.' In all relationships—our friendships, our family, our romantic relationships—love is in the action. Yet we expect ourselves to be able to look in the mirror and feel that love without doing any of the actions that feel loving. It doesn't make sense." If we have self-trust, then all of a sudden, we *believe* the words we're telling ourselves. They're not empty affirmations; they're laden with historic weight and meaning.

Self-trust is built by the same process as trust in any other relationship: it comes from keeping promises. If you kept making dates with your friend and she kept not showing up, your trust in her would wane. If your partner kept saying they were going to take the trash out but never did, would you believe them when they promise to clean the bathroom? Likely not. Yet we think there are no consequences when we break those promises to ourselves. When we say, *I'm going to wake up early today and meditate,* but hit the snooze button five times, when we vow we'll start that screenplay that's living in our brains but never sit to write the first sentence, when we promise our bodies nourishment but keep feeding them things that make us feel like crap: these are all broken promises, and they all erode self-trust. And then when you look in the mirror and say, "I love you" or "I believe in you" or "You can do this"—well, why would you believe that person? They've never stuck to their word before.

Today, make a promise to yourself. It doesn't need to be big—in fact, a huge mistake we often make when starting a new habit is to go too big. When we try to tackle too much, we set ourselves up for failures of self-trust (*of course* you're not going to be able to meditate for an hour every single day), which in turn leads to failures of self-love (*Why am I such a horrible person? I can't even do this one thing right*).

Instead, look for tiny opportunities to evidence that you keep the promises you make to yourself. Go for a walk around the block. Actually close your computer at a certain time. Meditate for five minutes, do a gratitude practice—you could even pick an action from one of the other pages of this book. But whatever you choose, commit to it. Show up for yourself so you can trust yourself, so that when you tell yourself you love yourself, you actually believe it.

38.

Eliminate jealousy.

I'm ruthless about unfollowing accounts on social media that make me feel bad about myself and blocking algorithmically generated content designed to push my buttons. It sounds easy and obvious enough, but so often we fail to pay attention to the pangs of jealousy, anger, sadness, and other negative emotions we experience when we're mindlessly scrolling. Maybe it's an ex you're following because you want to believe you're friends, but whose posts make you sting with loss. Maybe it's a high school friend you want to keep tabs on, but whose "perfect" photos make you feel like a failure. Maybe it's a celebrity who you think is inspiring you, but is actually making you resent the fact that your desk job is not, in fact, on a yacht in Ibiza.

There's a fine line between that which inspires and that which inspires resentment for our current situations, and the line isn't static; it needs to be constantly reevaluated. In the past, I negotiated myself into keeping people on my feed for *years* after I should've let them go. What if I need their tips? (Google is real, and you'll likely be able to find more expert sources.) What if I lose my motivation? (Feeling bad about ourselves is far less motivating than making changes from a place of self-love and respect.) What if they notice? Well—this one actually has merit in the case of family members or friends, but that's what the "mute" button was invented for.

Another sneaky way reality-warping perceptions permeate our brains is via the television we watch. Yes, all the reality shows with millionaires selling houses to other millionaires or wildly wealthy people catfighting are brain candy—but they also move our baseline for what a "normal" life looks like. We build our expectations, both conscious and subconscious, off our exposures. And if every week you're exposing yourself to hours and hours of people buying designer handbags, living in megamansions, and flying first class—well, is it surprising if your normal, beautiful life starts to feel less shiny? That envy for something you didn't even know you wanted would begin to creep in?

As famed psychologist Dr. Julie Smith shared with me, "We get trapped in this marketing frenzy that tells us if we can just have more, be more, do more, earn more, and then buy more, everything will be better. In my practice, I've worked with all kinds of people from all walks of life, and I can tell you this is not the case. It's just not." Maybe you don't get to hear the innermost secrets of some of the most successful people on the planet like Dr. Smith does, but we can all benefit from the same perspective shift.

Sometimes it's not strangers but people we're in *close* relationships with who spark that sting. Maybe a coworker gets a promotion you wanted, or a close friend sends pictures from a vacation you could never afford, captioned "I wish you were here."

In these scenarios, Dr. Smith said, it's ideal to turn that envy into information, then turn that information into inspiration. "If there's somebody that I envy, I ask myself, 'What is it I'm envious about? What is it I want that they have? Is it their job? Their relationship?' And then I ask: 'How have they achieved it?'" she said. "And if I really do want it, how can I move towards it?"

The key, Dr. Smith shared, is to get really curious and follow the chain of thought as far as you can, probing and asking yourself about the reasons behind your feelings. "If it is something you really want, then that person becomes someone you can learn from about how to move forward. You can look at how they've done it and see what you can learn from the experience." It can be helpful to truly take this step to its extreme and, as if you're a detective, pick apart whatever it is that the person has. What specific steps did they take? What jobs did they work previously that laddered up to the job they have? Where did they meet their partner? You can even role-play: If they were going to offer you one piece of advice to push your goals in the direction of their successes, what would it be?

If possible, I love to even take an opportunity to reach out to the person in question to ask some of my questions. It's a vulnerable experience but a powerful one, and you'll often find both valuable wisdom and a demystification of the shiny version of reality you're perceiving. Humanization is one of the most powerful tools we have in the face of envy, and after interviewing a lot of extremely wealthy, successful people, I can tell you assuredly that life on the other side of those dreams looks far different than we think.

If you find that you're envious about something you don't actually want, and the envy is just a symptom of a brain tending toward negative thought patterns, *or* you're envious about something that you'll never have access to (no matter what I do, I'll never be a supermodel, which makes my envy hard to use as inspiration), Dr. Smith suggested switching to gratitude. "Look at what you *do* have. If you're not satisfied with what you have, what is it you truly want instead? It's probably not a private jet or shiny hair. What are you actually missing, on a deeper level?" Maybe it's the feeling of being heard. Maybe it's love. Maybe it's more acclaim and praise for the work that you do. Maybe it's a moment to truly relax. Act like a child and relentlessly ask why, following the chain down until you get to the root of your deepest, truest desires. It's hard for envy and gratitude to coexist, and it's hard for false needs to stand up to self-aware probing.

Stop engaging in content that sparks negative emotions, and the next time you feel envious, don't push it away. Instead, lean in and gently begin to explore it. What is that envy telling you? And how can it serve the goals you have for your life?

39.

Make a personal
Bill of Rights.

Sometimes, when we find ourselves not feeling good on a day-to-day basis, it's because we're living by a set of unwritten rules that's not serving us. These rules are sneaky and ubiquitous: They start off as momentary acceptances to smooth the bumps in our work or home life. Then they happen again and again, and soon, we're pedestalizing other people's needs while ignoring our own, causing exhaustion, depression, and resentment.

To combat this, psychologist, bestselling *Not Nice* author, and Center for Social Confidence founder Dr. Aziz Gazipura shared a genius recommendation when I had him on an episode all about cultivating more confidence: creating a personal Bill of Rights. The list is composed of things you're giving yourself permission to do or feel—regardless of what your parents or society might have taught you. Start by taking a moment to really think about what you want your life to look like, outside of the *shoulds*. If you're getting stuck in the shoulds and having a hard time distancing yourself, it can be helpful to think about what you'd tell your best friend or child that they deserve. Would you tell them to constantly sacrifice their needs for the needs of others? Would you tell them to always take on the extra task at work, in lieu of spending quality time with the people or activities they love?

Once you make your Bill of Rights, treat it as a living document that you consult in times of decision, and add new rights as they spring up. The rights might feel abstract at first, but once you begin to apply them to specific situations in your life, you'll quickly become aware of all the micro-violations that have been taking place—and suddenly, it'll be blatantly obvious why you feel sluggish or sad or burnt out or any number of negative emotions. Your rights—that you do not have to earn, that you have simply by existing—are being violated moment to moment, hour to hour. Whether you're consciously aware of it or not, you're internalizing that breach, and there's no way that can't have an impact on your mental and physical being.

"Any single one of those rights can completely change your life," Dr. Gazipura explained. "Let's say, for example, one of your rights is 'I have a right to be treated with a certain level of respect,' and you find yourself in a conversation with someone who keeps talking over you. If you hadn't identified that right, you might just let it go, or *worse*, flip it on yourself, thinking, 'I shouldn't have upset them,' or 'Their ideas were more worth sharing.'" But with a Bill of Rights in place, you can immediately notice: *This is violating one of my rights.* "You'll have this whole other capacity to say, 'I can't keep having this conversation with you if you're going to keep doing this.' It gives you permission to let out a whole other version of yourself, because you need to protect your rights."

I'm not going to sugarcoat it: people might be disappointed by or upset with you. But this is one of the prices of authenticity. You can push toward the life of your dreams, a life that is wholly, fully *you*, or you can spend your life trying to be liked by everybody, a task at which you will certainly fail anyway.

I've included some sample rights—use them as jumping-off points to think about what *your* document might look like. Keep it on your phone. Read it regularly. Update it. Live by it. Give yourself the tools to grant yourself the respect you deserve from others—and, more important, from *yourself.*

SAMPLE RIGHTS

I have a right to feel any feeling.

I have a right to advocate for myself.

I have a right to say no.

I have a right to ask for what I want.

I have a right to ask again or make my case if someone says no to me.

I have a right to be treated with respect.

I have a right to like what I like without
knowing why or needing to explain it.

I have a right to dislike what I don't like without
knowing why or needing to explain it.

I have a right to challenge people.

I have a right to upset people.

I have a right to say no.

40.

Build belief in yourself.

Many of the experts I've interviewed cite a gratitude practice as a game changer for overall wellness. The practice has a strong scientific grounding because, as *New York Times* bestselling author and senior fellow at UC Berkeley's Greater Good Science Center Dr. Rick Hanson says, "Neurons that fire together, wire together" (for more on that, see page 152). When you fire your gratitude neurons, you prime them to fire more, and thus make yourself more likely to feel gratitude and other positive emotions in the future.

Dr. Tara Swart Bieber shared a new insight about gratitude practice that I hadn't heard before: "When I changed my gratitude journaling from things in my external life that I was grateful for to tools inside me that I was grateful for, it gave me a feeling of 'Whatever life throws at me next, I know that I have these resources to be able to deal with it better than I did the first time.'" Dr. Swart Bieber started this gratitude practice during her divorce, and she credits it with helping her build the resilience she needed to deal with the circumstances she was in at the time.

What if you're having trouble identifying positive qualities about yourself? "If you're already in a negative thought spiral, it can be really hard to suddenly say, 'I have resilience' and 'I have courage,'" said Dr. Swart Bieber. There are two tools that can help in this circumstance.

The first is identifying with a powerful icon. "Pick someone that you really admire. It might be an actress. It might be a historical figure. It might be someone in your life," said Dr. Swart Bieber. "Sit down and think about all the qualities that they possess that you really admire. And then just do a meditation where you embody those characteristics yourself."

According to Dr. Swart Bieber, this practice can make you realize that you yourself already have the qualities you admire. "And maybe you can see them in other people, but you can't see them in yourself," she said.

But it also works on a second level of proving to ourselves that those qualities are possible. As humans, we have a very hard time imagining things that we haven't seen demonstrated to be possible. One oft-cited, powerful example is the four-minute mile: Humans didn't believe it was possible to run that fast. But after one person managed to pull it off, several other people ran four-minute miles in quick succession.[1] Similarly, identifying these role models demonstrates to your brain that the traits you want to embody, the things you want to achieve, are possible. You can even reach for proof points in your own brain.

"Maybe you've already achieved something similar," Dr. Swart Bieber said, "so you can keep reminding yourself, 'I did *that*, so I can do *this*.'"

The second tool is to physically take care of yourself. Dr. Swart Bieber was quick to point out that believing in ourselves isn't entirely a mental practice (she is, after all, an MD in addition to having a PhD in neuroscience!). "If your brain is in a good environment, you're less likely to think negatively," she said. "If you skipped meals, if you didn't sleep much last night, you're going to be more likely to think, 'Oh, that's never gonna happen for me,' or 'I'm not as smart.' But when you're in the best possible physical state, then you could sit down and do that meditation and feel like, 'Yeah, actually, I have those qualities. Maybe not all of them, but I have some of them already.'" This is similar to the view held by Dr. Ellen Vora, Yale- and Columbia-trained board-certified psychiatrist and author of *The Anatomy of Anxiety*, that identifying "false moods" is one of the key aspects of managing our mental health (see page 258). While there is a tendency to view our minds as separate and distinct from more body-based elements of health like our hormones and sleep and blood sugar, in fact, all the parts are intrinsically entangled. I view this not as a negative, but as a beautiful method of permission giving for those days when we aren't great at loving ourselves, which will inevitably still come, regardless of our practices. Instead of attributing the negative feeling to something being intangibly, unchangeably "wrong" with you, maybe you can poke into your physical state a bit: Are you well-hydrated? Are you well-fed? How would it feel to sleep for a night and self-reflect again in the morning *before* you decide definitively that you're a worthless human being? Sometimes, self-love is an inside-out job, and sometimes, it's an outside-in one.

Approach loving yourself not as an esoteric goal but as a practice, with neuroscientific tools at your disposal to help make it a reality.

41.

Unlock the hidden information in your emotions.

We all know we're supposed to be living according to our values. But in a world with so much outside noise, it can be hard to discern what those values actually are. Dr. Susan David, an award-winning Harvard psychologist and author of *Emotional Agility*, has a solution.

When I spoke with Dr. David, she suggested that as a society, we're not dealing with our emotions in the ideal way. Not only are we often pushing down the emotions we have, we're not recognizing them as the vital information sources they are. When correctly grappled with, our emotions can tell us who we are and what we value in this world.

The first step is to stop shaming yourself for having emotions in the first place, a process that not only is self-harming, but also bluntly stops our ability to extract information from said emotions. Dr. David explains: "A type one emotion is where you feel the feeling—you feel sad, or grieving, or angry. Type two is when we start layering on whether we can, can't, should, or shouldn't experience a difficult emotion." This could look like feeling unhappy in your job, but then telling yourself you should be grateful because at least you have a job. It could look like feeling sad and then judging yourself for your sadness—after all, so many people have it so much worse. It's a sunny day! You're well-fed! Why can't you just be happy? It might look like growing up in a family that says, "We don't do anger here."

"One of the very first ways that we begin to develop our emotional agility is by recognizing that every single emotional experience that we have had and will ever have in our lives is actually part of our evolutionary, adaptive system," Dr. David said. "When you feel a difficult emotion, that emotion is often signposting that there's a value that's being threatened, a need that's unmet, or something else that's important to you that's become really critical. A very important first part of emotional agility is what I call 'gentle acceptance' in my work."

Simply put—your emotions are not only valid, but a critical part of your survival in this world. They're not embarrassing or selfish or impolite. Picture your emotions as messages from your innermost self. You can either crumple up the paper and throw it aside ("I don't have time for this! You don't deserve to send a message through right now!"), or you can read the message and use it to inform your next steps.

Dr. David explained that gentle noticing is the key to gentle acceptance: "Gentle noticing looks like: 'I'm noticing that I'm feeling really depleted. I'm noticing my grief. I'm noticing my sadness, my loneliness.' When you notice your inner world with a level of compassion and gentleness, you are no longer in the type two emotion, where you're fighting against your emotional experience, and instead you're just able to be with it. And when you can be with your emotional experience, it defangs that emotional experience automatically."

Moreover, noticing the emotion can help you actually begin to discover what your values are. "The experience of loneliness is heartbreaking, and common. We can be lonely in a room full of people," said Dr. David. "That loneliness is often signposting that you need more intimacy and connection. Boredom is signposting that you value learning and growth; you need more of it. Grief is love looking for its home. When I experience these moments being sucked into grief, instead of racing for the exits, I recognize that that grief is often saying, 'See me. Remember me. Connect with those memories. Connect with the things that I gave you.' There's something really powerful in that."

Difficult emotions aren't just things that we need to tolerate, but rather data that's flagging our needs and our values. And when we sit with, explore, and accept those difficult emotions, we're no longer driven by them. Instead, they become important information to power the journey to where *we* want to go.

The next time you feel an emotion, don't layer judgment on top of it. Instead, simply notice it. Try to acknowledge and accept it, and then ask what it might be trying to give you. Your emotions are not only valid, they are critical messages that you can use to identify your true inner desires and necessities. Judging or ignoring that information just pulls you further away from living your most authentic and fully-realized life.

42.

Learn to love your body.

One of the most popular series on the podcast is called "How I Learned to Love My Body," which is about real people sharing their journey to, well, loving their body. I intentionally don't use the phrase "body positivity," which was initially created to help promote the acceptance of marginalized bodies, and has since been co-opted by many people in nonmarginalized bodies and dominant social groups. I also don't want people to have a toxically positive relationship with their body, insisting that they need to find it "beautiful" or consider themselves "pretty." This sentiment, while on the surface compelling, still puts looking a certain way at the top of the pedestal. Why is something aesthetically focused even the goal?

Instead, I use the word "love." Love is a complicated relationship. Love goes through ups and downs. Love doesn't always mean *like*. What love is, and the relationship that I hope you and I and every other person on this planet get to someday have with our bodies, is deep and abiding commitment, appreciation, and respect. You do not need to think you have attractive thighs to love your body. You don't need to enjoy how it appears in any way, as a matter of fact, because your body is for *living*, not looking. You do need to accept, however, that this is the body you've got, and figure out what you want this lifelong relationship to be. The series is all about real people navigating that question, and sharing what they learned along the way.

One of my guests, Hunter McGrady, is a bona fide supermodel, having appeared in the *Sports Illustrated* Swimsuit Issue a whopping five times. She wasn't, however, born with the type of confidence that lets someone pose in a tiny bikini knowing millions of people will see the photos—or, in Hunter's case the very first time she worked with the magazine, pose for photos completely naked, aside from a swimsuit made of paint.

Hunter's relationship with her body has been crafted and earned over time, and in our conversation, she shared one of her top secrets for learning to love her body. "My therapist told me about this exercise. She said, 'The next time you shower, I want you to strip any makeup, anything off of you. Get down to your bare self, then look in the mirror and say five things that you love about yourself. And if you can't find things you love about yourself, I want you to say things you want to love.'" Hunter tried the exercise and had a really hard time with it. "I started crying. And I just thought, 'What is the point of this? I hate it.' And I came back and my therapist was like, 'How was it?' And I said, 'Well, it wasn't great, to be honest with you.'" Great, Hunter's therapist said—now I want you to do that every single time you shower. "So I did," said Hunter. "And soon enough, after enough times, the things that I wanted to love about myself ended up being the things that I loved about myself. And those things grew and grew and grew and grew. And instead of five things, it was ten things. And then ten became twenty. And then the things moved from the physical to inner stuff, to the things that make me *me*. And now, thirteen years later, I still do this exercise."

If you think about it, in our lives, we've heard literally thousands, maybe hundreds of thousands of times what not to love about our bodies. There are billion-dollar industries predicated on the fact that we think our thighs are too small or too large, or that our skin should be unlined, poreless, and blemish-free. To even begin to tip the scales toward feeling satisfied with who we are, we need to pile on some messages that come from a far more loving place—especially messages directed at our literally most revealed, stripped-bare selves. It's okay if you don't believe what you're saying at the beginning: there was probably a time you didn't believe society's messages, either, but repetition has a way of infiltrating our brains. "It's going to feel totally fake at first," Hunter said. "It's going to feel really awkward and weird and uncomfortable. But just follow through with it for a couple of months. Try it every day. I think you're going to see a really, really big change."

A FEW THINGS THAT HAVE HELPED ME CHANGE MY RELATIONSHIP WITH MY BODY

1. The single biggest game changer for me has been shifting my focus from how my body *looks* to how it *feels* (see page 17). At the gym, I don't lift my shirt to check the appearance of my abs in the mirror; I focus on how good it feels to be sore, how my anxiety has dissipated, how powerful I feel. When I eat, I don't think about how the food will impact my hips or thighs; I focus on how satiated I feel, how delicious the flavors were, and how I feel sharper, focused, and more ready to take on the day.

2. I'm incredibly conscious of whom I follow on social media, and regularly go on sprees where I unfollow literally hundreds of people at a time. I used to think that seeing these bodies was inspiring me, but the insidious messaging of social media and other types of media seeps into our brains and gives us false impressions of what our lives and bodies should look like (see page 125). Schedule time once a month to curate your feeds so you're only taking in content that makes you feel good.

3. When someone I'm in conversation with starts talking negatively about bodies (either mine, their own, or culturally), I gently but firmly request that we change the subject to something more interesting.

4. I started wearing clothes that I loved and that made me feel good. As one of my favorite podcast guests, personal stylist Charly Goss, always said, "F*ck flattering." Even the concept of flattering is based on manipulating your body toward an "ideal" body type dictated by someone else. And while we're on the subject, sizes are largely arbitrary and differ wildly from brand to brand. Buy clothes that *fit*; don't let a little fabric tag stand between you and your best life.

5. Thinking about my deathbed, per page 11, has been immensely helpful for making the place my body's appearance holds in my

consciousness feel more right-size. At the end of your life, are you going to be thinking, *Wow, my cellulite was so off-putting in that swimsuit*, or are you going to be thinking, *I can't believe I let a few ripples in my skin dictate the joy I felt on a beach*? Our time on this earth is limited. How sad to waste it focusing on things that, at the end of the day, will truly feel so insignificant.

6. I remember that around the world, there are so many types of bodies and faces that are considered beautiful, and how much our view of beauty has changed throughout history. Zooming out and realizing that the trends will continue to cycle and I'll never be able to succeed in all of them (how could I when they often actively contradict each other?) helps me to gently remove myself from the race.

7. A lot of product marketers and, frankly, social media influencers soft promise that if you buy what they sell or do what they do, your body will look like theirs. I was far, far too late in life when I realized this simply isn't true. I don't wake up every day thinking I'll go from 5'2" to 5'6" if I just put in enough effort. Why do I think the rest of my body will drastically change shape? Yes, we can add muscle and lose weight—to an extent. But realizing that, by and large, our bodies are our bodies and they'll *never* be anyone else's bodies—regardless of what we consume, or how many squats we do—is incredibly important and freeing. It leaves space to make our unique bodies feel as good as they possibly can, without trying to change them into someone else's.

8. I realized that I was trying to make my body look a certain way to be viewed better by other people—but when I think about the people I love, their looks rarely even factor into the equation. When you think about your friends or family members, does your mind go to the size of their stomach or their stretch marks? Do you think, *Wow, I'd enjoy this game night way more if they weighed five pounds less*? Or do you think about the way they make you laugh, their cooking skills, how empathetic they are when your life is rocky? Right. That's how other people are thinking about you.

9. My all-time favorite mantra: "My body is for living, not looking." It's for cuddling my cat, flooding me with pleasure, enjoying a favorite book, traveling to places that fill me with awe, laughing with my friends until my stomach hurts. My body is the vessel through which I experience life, not the lens through which people experience me. It was not made to serve as eye candy for other people, particularly when that comes at the detriment of my own experience. It was made to allow me to *live*.

WANT TO DIVE DEEPER?

Listen to these episodes of **The Liz Moody Podcast:**

- "How to Eliminate Jealousy, Build Self Love, and Feel More Satisfied with Your Life TODAY," episode 97
- "How to Become More Confident: Quiet Your Inner Critic, Stop People Pleasing, and Unlock a Bigger Life with Dr. Aziz Gazipura," episode 163
- The "How I Learned to Love My Body" series, with episodes featuring Hunter McGrady, Katie Sturino, Raeann Langas & Kristina Zias, Britney Vest, Achieng Agutu, and Victoria Browne

Explore these resources from our expert guests:

- *Radically Content: Being Satisfied in an Endlessly Dissatisfied World* by Jamie Varon, @jamievaron on Instagram
- *Not Nice: Stop People Pleasing, Staying Silent, & Feeling Guilty . . . and Start Speaking Up, Saying No, Asking Boldly, and Unapologetically Being Yourself* by Dr. Aziz Gazipura, www.draziz.com
- Hunter McGrady, @HunterMcGrady on Instagram

HOW TO
BE HAPPIER

43.

Make your schedule match your values.

One of the first questions positive psychologist Dr. Samantha Boardman asks clients when they visit her practice is: "What are the three things that you value most in your life?" It's a task that's more challenging than one might expect in a world where we're constantly told by society, authority figures, and even our own family members what our values should be. We're given so little room to reflect on *what* we value that it's not surprising that many of us don't even know where to begin when faced with that question.

It's a common problem, and Dr. Boardman has prompts designed to help suss out *your* unique values—not your mom's, not your boss's, not that influencer you follow on social media's, but *yours*. After clients write down their answer, she has them think about how they're spending their time, and especially their free time. What do they do on a Saturday or Sunday? What about after work?

I'm personally guilty of often feeling like my values aren't reflected in my days. In my interview with famed psychologist Dr. Rick Hanson about how to be happier, he invited me to spend one week tracking how I used my time. He suggested creating a spreadsheet or document (there are also apps that serve the same function, if you prefer!) with columns for each type of activity that makes up my day: sleeping, personal hygiene, getting dressed, eating, exercising, working, scrolling social media, reading the news, watching TV. Every fifteen minutes, for one week, I was to notate how I'd used the previous fifteen minutes.

"Don't change what you do," Dr. Hanson said. "Just tell the truth about how you spend your time."

Everyone he knows who has done this exercise, he shared, has had their mind blown. Tracking their activity revealed a lot of stuff they already knew, and it reassured them about some things they were worried about—maybe they get more done in a day than they thought, or had more social connection than they thought.

"But also, they always flag something really big," he said. "They realize, 'Wow! I'm spending about three and a half hours a day on absolute bullshit.' And you start to realize that your life could be so much better if you took at least *some* of that wasted time and applied it to doing the things that matter to you."

The exercise invites us not only to confront how we're using our time, but to reflect on the way we'd like to spend our days, and consider the factors getting in the way of those desires.

After realizing I spent far more time than I'd like on social media, I started keeping my phone out of the bedroom at night (see page 43) and setting app limits. I also started adding the things I *did* value to my calendar. When we put things into our calendar, we give them priority in our lives. And when we consistently add nothing but work tasks to our calendar—well, it's not a surprise that the work tasks get accomplished, often at the expense of our relationships with others, and with ourselves. My entire life changed when I started to add my personal goals to my calendar. I'll put a recurring meeting on my calendar to call my mom, or pencil in a five-minute block to text a friend to check in. I have date nights with Zack on my calendar, blocks to drink a smoothie with him outside before a long day, and quarterly finance check-ins.

Beyond that, I also schedule in my commitments to myself. Meditation goes in the calendar, along with daily workouts. My beloved circ walk (see page 33)? In the calendar. My workouts? In the calendar. Even time to *relax*, to read a book and just chill—it goes on the calendar and not just in the leftover space from my many to-dos. My rest is a priority, key to my mental health and enjoyment of life, and as necessary to my productivity as my moments of go-go-go. If I can take a break another time, great. But putting it in the calendar ensures that it will happen at least at the minimum of what I'm okay with.

The way we spend our hours turns into the way we spend our days, which turns into the way we spend our years. While some shifts toward your ideal life will take longer to make than others, they need to come from a place of being informed, and spending a week (or even a few days!) tracking your time is the first step toward creating that self-awareness. That way, you can make decisions rooted in evidence rather than speculation. Once you figure out how you're spending your time, you begin to shift your schedule to align it with your values.

44.

Build tolerance for hard things.

If you've ever felt numb to the simple pleasures of life, or like you have a hard time staying away from the temptations of your phone, drugs, alcohol, or other addictive substances, you might have an imbalance of dopamine,[1] the neurochemical responsible for motivation.

Dr. Anna Lembke, chief of the Stanford University Addiction Medicine Dual Diagnosis Clinic and author of *Dopamine Nation*, explained: "In our modern ecosystem, we're all constantly bombarding our reward pathway [in our brains] with these highly reinforcing, very potent drugs that come in almost any form—in our food, on the internet, in actual drugs that we take, both prescribed and otherwise—such that we've effectively changed our set point for experiencing pleasure and pain to a place where it's that much easier to experience pain, and we need a whole lot *more* pleasure to experience pleasure."

Dr. Lembke explained that the best way to grasp how dopamine works in our brain is to picture balancing a teeter-totter. "When we experience pleasure, it tips to one side, and when we experience pain, it tips to the opposite side," she said. The goal is to have the teeter-totter evenly balanced.

"There are three rules governing this balance," Dr. Lembke shared. "The first rule is that for every pleasure, we pay a price, because the way that the balance goes back to the neutral position is by tipping an equal amount to the opposite side of whatever the initial stimulus was."

Essentially, we're paying for our pleasures (especially simple dopamine spikes) with some kind of pain, such as the pain of craving more of that pleasure (more chocolate, more screen time). Other universal symptoms of a pleasure-pain balance tipped to the pain side include anxiety, irritability, insomnia, and dysphoria, or depressed moods.

"The second rule is probably the most important one for understanding how we get addicted," Dr. Lembke explained. "With repeated exposure to the same or similar stimulus, that initial response, the tilt to the side of pleasure, gets weaker and shorter, but that after response gets stronger and longer."

This is essentially what happens with addiction—the pleasure/pain set point changes and people need their drug of choice not only to feel *good*, but simply to restore a level of balance and feel *normal*.

"When people with substance use disorder are not using their drug of choice, their balance tips to the side of pain," Dr. Lembke said. "They're in a dopamine-deficit state, so they're irritable, anxious, craving, and narrowly focused on their drug." If you feel irritable when you don't have access to your phone, but you need more dopamine hits when you're *on* your phone—faster scrolling, more stimulation—this rule might feel familiar to you.

"The third rule is that we have an incredibly keen memory for that initial stimulus of either pleasure or pain," Dr. Lembke said. "You can imagine from an evolutionary perspective why that would be—we need to remember where that food source is, or where the lion's den is and that the last time, the lion nearly killed us, so that we don't go in that direction again." The problem is that our memory isn't nearly as good for the aftereffect, or the opponent process effect from rule one. So we might remember that first delicious bite of chocolate, but we don't remember irritably craving more and more of it, and needing more and more to be satisfied. Or we remember that blast of dopamine from opening our phone or drinking alcohol, but we don't remember the tech or booze hangover that inevitably comes after.

The secret to balancing your dopamine is, first and foremost, to moderate and in some cases completely avoid your drug of choice. But, interestingly, you also want to *intentionally invite painful experiences into your life.*

"By using mild to moderate noxious stimuli, we signal to the brain and the body that there's an injury, which causes them then to up-regulate production of our own endogenous feel-good neurotransmitters and hormones like dopamine, serotonin, and norepinephrine, our endocannabinoid system or endo-opioid system," explained Dr. Lembke.

Dr. Lembke suggested incorporating stressors like vigorous exercise, cold showers (see page 64 for more on that), and cognitively challenging tasks that provoke frustration, like reading a difficult book or solving a tricky puzzle. "In this day and age, just unplugging for a while and tolerating boredom and silence can be plenty distressing, because we're so used to the constant stimulation," she said. "The neat thing about these kinds of activities is that there's not a dopamine spike followed by a dopamine plunge, but rather a gradual, slow increase of dopamine as we progress in the activity, which then remains elevated for hours afterwards."

Dr. Lembke said the natural challenges that life throws at us can also be viewed constructively in this context—for instance, getting caught in the rain laden with heavy grocery bags becomes not simply a frustration, but a dopamine-balancing experience.

"In that moment of doing the hard thing, you're basically producing dopamine," Dr. Lembke said. "It reframes that experience to be instead of 'Poor me, this is really hard, this is really unpleasant' to something like, 'Wow, this is really good for me. And this is going to pay off dividends going forward.' It becomes like a project you want to do."

Look for opportunities to gently press on the pain side of the teeter-totter, whether you're taking a cold shower or reading a challenging book. But also use this science to help shift your mindset around the challenging moments that naturally occur in your life, as they do for all of us. Those feelings of difficulty are increasing your ability to motivate yourself, avoid dopamine-spiking temptations, and derive pleasure from simpler activities in the future.

In those moments of challenge, while it can be tempting to reach for your phone, a drink, or another dopamine-spiking self-soother and let those gremlins hop on the other side of the teeter-totter, you want to instead build tolerance for the challenge, for the frustration. Whether you chose the challenge or not, it's serving as a positive investment in your neurochemistry.

45.

Rewire your neural pathways for happiness.

If there was ever an episode of my podcast that feels like a warm hug, it's "Ask the Doctor: Happiness Edition." Psychologist Dr. Rick Hanson has spent his career studying what makes us really, truly happy on our deepest levels, and the wisdom he shares incorporates everything from Zen Buddhism to the latest neuroscience.

Neuroplasticity, or the brain's ability to change and adapt over time, is one of the most exciting areas of his research. Simply put, it means that our brains aren't fixed; rather, our neural pathways literally change over time. And the craziest part is? A lot of it is in our control.

Picture your brain like a field. When you think a thought or engage in a behavior, you walk through the field. When you *rethink* that thought or redo that behavior, you rewalk that same path. When you think a different thought or engage in a different behavior, you walk a different path. Over time, certain paths will become well-trod, easy to spot with their worn-down grass, while others might grow over and become difficult to bushwhack through. Our brains want the easy route: they'll opt for the well-trod path.

The key, then, to intentionally wire your brain to feel more happiness, is to *walk the paths of happiness*. You want these to be the most well-worn routes in your brain. You want your brain to think,

That trail? I can do it with my eyes closed. I know it like the back of my hand.

In our interview, Dr. Hanson shared one of the most simple and effective ways to build those pathways: notice the good feelings throughout your daily life and linger in those feelings for slightly longer than you might otherwise.

This can be as simple as looking out the window and noticing an interesting bird, sinking into a snuggle with a child or pet or partner, feeling the sunlight warming your skin, or biting into a ripe, juicy piece of fruit. Whatever the positive feeling is, notice it, then linger in it. By noticing and lingering, you're strengthening the neural pathways in your brain that are designed to help you feel good,[1] even in the moments you're *not specifically trying to.* By strengthening those pathways, you're making your brain *more likely to take them.* Meaning, your brain will *choose* to feel good at more moments in the future because you've trained those neurons to wire together.

This is one of my favorite tips in this book because you don't have to devote any special period of time to it—rather, it just fits into the course of your normal life, *and* it has ripple effects that extend far beyond the moment or two within which you're practicing it. It's literally a way to harness what we know about neuroscience to feel happier on a daily basis—and not in a rah-rah, toxic way, but rather on a concrete, *physiological* level.

Look out for good feelings, tiny and large. And when you notice them, linger on them. Count to five. Take in the sensations. And know that little by little, you're building a brain that will support you, that will fill you with good feelings, that will help you live *your* best life, every single day.

46.

Do something for someone else.

If you've been on a plane, you've heard a flight attendant say, "Put on your own mask before helping someone near you." The adage has become somewhat of a mantra for self-care (along with the frequently used "how can you pour from an empty cup?"), and in general, it's something I applaud.

But also.

There are moments when the best thing you can do to fill your cup *is* to fill someone else's. When I interviewed positive psychiatrist Dr. Samantha Boardman, she shared that one of her favorite ways to alleviate stress and burnout is to be of value to another person. "Interestingly, when you actually do something for another person, you feel a *restored* sense of time," she said. "Instead of that time famine that you're probably experiencing, you get a time feast. It also creates a sense of self-efficacy, because you're affirmed in your capability of contributing to someone else's life."[1]

Another reason this works, explained Dr. Boardman, is that it gets us out of our own heads. "We're often told to focus on ourselves. 'How am I feeling? What's going on in my brain?' It can take us into this place of self-immersion, and self-immersion often ends up with rumination." Rumination is a process that involves thinking about the same thought or event over and over, and abundant research associates it strongly with depression.[2] Too much self-focus, then, isn't actually helping us; it's leading us to feel *worse*. Doing good for others promotes a sense of belonging and a feeling of community, and reinforces the social bonds that are so critical to our happiness (see page 179).

While this book is filled with ideas to explore your own head and strap on your oxygen mask, I recommend doing one thing for another person today, and exploring how it makes you feel. I've included a list of ideas here, but lean into anything that resonates.

- Call a friend and ask about what's going on in their life.

- Offer to run an errand or pick up groceries for a neighbor.

- Call a local organization and ask how you can help.

- Donate money to a cause you believe in.

- Ask any new parents, people who are ill, or elderly people in your life if you can drop off a homemade meal for them.

- Teach someone a useful skill that you have.

- Call your parents or parental figures and ask if there's anything you can help them with.

- Do a household chore that your partner appreciates but has been avoiding.

- Give someone you love a five-minute hand or shoulder massage.

- Make a care package and send it to someone in another city.

- Offer to babysit so a parent in your life can enjoy a night out.

- Text someone to tell them why you love or appreciate them.

47.

Fill your life with joy.

I went into my interview with Catherine Price, author of *The Power of Fun*, expecting her to offer a prescription for how to have more fun every single day. And while she did share some tricks for that, what she impressed upon me even more was that fun is *already happening*—we simply need to attune ourselves to its presence.

One way that Price finds the fun in her life is engaging in something she calls a delights practice, which she was inspired to adopt by Ross Gay's *The Book of Delights*. The idea is that our lives are actually filled with delights, but because we don't practice seeing them, many of them slip by without us noticing them. There's a psychological phenomenon called the frequency illusion, wherein after you draw your attention to something, you begin to notice it everywhere. While the thing doesn't *actually* increase in frequency, it appears to, because suddenly your attention is attuned to it. You can take advantage of this phenomenon by intentionally noticing what you want your brain to notice *more* of. When you start seeking out delight, you'll suddenly find it everywhere.

You can start by simply noting the delight, and even saying the word "delight" aloud. Price actually wears a bracelet that reads *Delight* that she had made to remind herself of the practice. She also recommends amplifying the effects of the practice by sharing it with a friend—Price has a delights text chain. "I have a friend I reconnected with a couple years ago from college, and he texted me a photo last winter of his windshield with frost on it. And it said,

'Delight,'" Price shared. "And I love that as an example, because he had a choice there. It was either a really annoying thing, because he's on his way to work and he had to clean his windshield from frost, or he had the choice to notice the delight in the beauty of the frost crystal and think, 'I'm going to share it with my friend Catherine.' And he chose the latter, and I got delight from his delight, which made me want to look for more delight. It sparked a whole delight cycle."

In addition to keeping an eye out for delights that spring up, you can also create a "Joy List" to identify the things that light you up, so you can intentionally fill your life with more of them. Start by making a list of experiences from the recent or more distant past that stand out to you as having felt incredibly positive. Who were you with? What were you doing? Where were you? Once you have a list of three to five moments, start to look for themes. Are there certain friends you always have a blast with? Experiences that always make you feel good? Places that consistently light you up? What are the common denominators in your "fun"?

I have to confess: making this list was initially a struggle for me. I had spent years working early mornings and late nights, spending my burnt-out time off scrolling through social media, deriving tiny hits of dopamine and little in the way of real pleasure. I was so involved in becoming, working toward a far-off future when joy would come effortlessly, that I had forgotten how to truly *be*.

And then I started paying attention. That instant calm that flooded my body when I lay on the floor and put my legs up a wall? Joy. Brewing a pot of my favorite tea? Joy. Singing along with tens of thousands of people at a Taylor Swift concert? Joy. The more joy I noticed, the more joy seemed to exist (because I was building neural pathways that were primed toward happiness, as Dr. Rick Hanson taught us on page 152). I began to use my Joy List to dictate the experiences I prioritized—concerts are a more regular occurrence, I try to put my legs up the wall before bed every night, and hikes have become a weekly nonnegotiable. And the more joy that exists in my present, the less pressure I feel to sacrifice this moment for a future that might never come.

Tuning into my actual joy also put into stark contrast the parts of my life that were actually coping or dissociating mechanisms disguised as joy. Many of the activities we label as "self-care" actually make us feel worse afterward and rob us of time for true joy in the long run. For me, that's watching reality TV and scrolling social media for hours. It's like eating cotton candy: it feels good for a second, but then dissolves completely, leaving me with a vague ache where the sweet once was. Don't add things to your Joy List if you do them to "zone out" or "turn off"—the goal is joy, not escapism.

We don't live in a world that prioritizes fun (despite the many health benefits that Price noted in our interview, including lower stress levels,[1] decreased risk of illness,[2] and increased longevity[3]). Whether you start a delights practice or take ten minutes to brainstorm a Joy List, it's time to start seeking out—and prioritizing—the fun in your life.

48.

Make a "Life Is Never Boring" list.

Look, we all know life isn't boring. We *know* it. But sometimes, when you finally get a window of free time, it can be hard to think of what to actually do with it. When I spoke with Olivia Amitrano, founder of modern herbal medicine company Organic Olivia, she shared one of her antidotes to this: the "Life Is Never Boring" list. "Whenever I have a moment where I'm like, 'This would be such a good opportunity for self-care, but nothing's coming to mind right now,' or 'I'm too overwhelmed. I have decision fatigue, I don't know what to do,' I open up a list I keep on my phone that details everything I can do in all of those little moments that I know will make me feel juicy or cared for," she explained.

Renowned Yale professor and happiness psychologist Dr. Laurie Santos has lauded a similar concept, which she calls a "time confetti to-do list." Time confetti references small windows of time we have between meetings or when we're waiting for a train to come or a pot to boil. We often spend those moments on social media, which leads to us feeling time starved—we never have enough time to do what we truly value, because even in those tiny slivers of time we do have, we're essentially eating the equivalent of time junk food. Dr. Santos argues that we'd feel much more satisfied if we used those small blocks for things we actually find satisfying and, because those things are so hard to pluck from thin air in the moment, that we have a list ready to go that we can consult when an opportunity arises.

I made my own time confetti to-do/Life Is Never Boring list after interviewing Amitrano. The process couldn't have been simpler; I pulled up a notes app on my phone and started listing things that brought me satisfaction or pleasure and fit into increments from fractional (a minute or two) to much larger (an hour or more).

If you're looking for some thought starters for your own list, I've shared some items from my own here. But your list is your own, so ask yourself: How do you wish you used your time? And then when you find yourself in one of those moments, instead of scrolling social media, open your notes app and pick something from the list. Use your time windows to create the life you want to live.

- Text a friend, especially someone I've been meaning to get back to or in touch with but haven't.

- Cuddle my cat, Bella.

- Paint my nails.

- Go for a five-minute walk outside.

- Call a family member.

- Download a language app and practice a few sentences.

- Delete emails.

- Put on a song I love and dance wildly.

- Squeeze lemons or blend fresh ginger with water and pour it into an ice cube tray for the best warm drinks later.

- Start planning my next vacation.

- Google upcoming shows of my favorite artists/venues so I don't miss any I love.

- Prep some veggies to have on hand in the fridge so they're easier to eat later.

- Stretch.

- Drink a big glass of water.

- Organize my pantry.

- Put on a podcast, even if it's just for five minutes.

- Add friends' birthdays to my Google Calendar as recurring annual events.

- Write out a grocery list.

- Do four rounds of box breathing (page 261).

- Make that doctor/dentist appointment I've been stalling on.

- Carry around a book with short, digestible segments (like this one!) so I can sneak in five-minute reading chunks.

- Write down a big dream for the future and one way to propel myself toward it.

- Make a cup of tea.

WANT TO DIVE DEEPER?

Listen to these episodes of The Liz Moody Podcast:

- "Ask the Doctor: Happiness Edition—How to Feel More Content & at Peace, Regardless of Your Life Circumstances with Dr. Rick Hanson, PhD," episode 69

- "How to Hack Your Dopamine to Stop Reaching for Your Phone and Experience More Pleasure in Everyday Life with Dr. Anna Lembke," episode 98

- "Ask the Doctor: Stress Edition—Exactly How to Identify and

Eliminate Stress in Your Life with Dr. Samantha Boardman,"
episode 78

Explore these resources from our expert guests:

- *Neurodharma: New Science, Ancient Wisdom, and Seven Practices of the Highest Happiness* by Dr. Rick Hanson, www .RickHanson.net

- *Dopamine Nation: Finding Balance in the Age of Indulgence* by Dr. Anna Lembke, www.annalembke.com

- *Everyday Vitality: Turning Stress into Strength* by Dr. Samantha Boardman, @drsamanthaboardman on Instagram

HOW TO MAKE AND KEEP FRIENDS

49.

Attract your dream friends.

There's the old adage that we are the average of the five people we hang out with the most, and whether or not you agree with the specific number, there's no doubt that the people we surround ourselves with have a huge impact on the people we are and the directions in which we grow. Yet often, we fall into relationships of convenience—friends from high school or college, people who happened to be on our team at work, spouses of our spouse's friends. If our friends are molding us in conscious and subconscious ways, one of the most effective ways to spur our own evolution is to be intentional about who those people are. If you find yourself looking around at the people you spend the most time with and thinking, *Wait, this doesn't reflect my values,* or *This is encouraging a contracted mindset, not an expansive one,* but you don't know what to do *next,* bestselling author Tara Schuster has you covered.

"The first thing is writing down what you want," Schuster explained. "Be as specific as possible. 'People who lift me up.' 'People who have interesting and inspiring hobbies.' 'People I always feel energized after spending time with.' 'People who have cool careers that I can learn from.' Write as much as possible."

Having specificity both allows us to have direction, and allows us to reprogram the stories we're telling ourselves about the type of person we are, the types of people we're worthy of attracting, and the type of life we're capable of having. Don't limit yourself—just write it all down.

Now survey the landscape of your social situation. "Look at the people you currently know and ask, 'Are my nearest and dearest doing these things? Are they meeting these needs?'" Schuster said. "Sometimes you'll see that within your group, there might be people you're spending a lot of time with who are actually sucking you dry. Learning to let go of people who you've outgrown or you've just diverged paths with—that's not a bad thing. It's actually natural. It's growth. And maybe you'll come back together one day in the future, but you definitely won't if you continue on this negative path."

You don't need to be explicit about a friendship breakup. If the idea of having a "talk" gives you palpitations, you can simply move that person into a different category in your life. Maybe they are now just the person you go to yoga classes with. Maybe they're a person you text with occasionally instead of talking to for hours about the problems in your lives. Drawing the boundary and explicitly defining the desired relationship in your head is the most important part; whether you want to express this to the other person is completely up to you, and is dependent on the particular relationship you have with that person.

The next step is to start to fill in your newly opened spaces with the types of people you want to surround yourself with, who meet the criteria you defined in the first part of the exercise. The best way to do that, Schuster said, is by casting a wider net toward the people who already exist in your life. "Look at your orbit of acquaintances," Schuster said. "Is there anybody in that circle who kind of matches what you're looking for? I personally did this recently. I knew I wanted to grow my circle of friends. I wrote down what I was looking for—for me, it was that I wanted to be going down a more spiritual path. I wanted to meet people whose number one value was kindness over everything else. Then I looked at the acquaintances I had to see if there was anybody in that group who kind of fit that criteria, and one woman did. I reached out to her and told her all of the specific things I admired about her. And then I just asked, 'Would you be open to doing some calls? Can we talk more often?' She lives across the country from me, but since then, we've been talking more often and building a stronger bond. And now I'm doing a virtual meditation retreat with her next week."

Is there anyone in your life who fits your criteria, whom you could begin to form a deeper relationship with? And if not, where can you go where you can start to expose yourself to these types of people? Where would a person who embodies the traits you've identified spend their time?

You're not too late. You're not too old. Everyone doesn't already have their friends. People are growing and changing all of the time, and their needs for their social dynamics change right along with them.

PS: After talking to Schuster, I identified her as someone who embodied a lot of the traits I was hoping to fill my friendship circle with. I told her as much, and invited her on a hike when she was traveling near me. Now she's one of my favorite people to talk to. The strategy works!

50.

Take advantage of the mere exposure effect.

If you're anything like me, you've probably thought fondly back to your school years, when making a new best friend was as easy as being assigned to the desk next to theirs in third period. As it turns out, science can help us understand why making friends was so easy back then yet feels so difficult now—and we can use that knowledge to hack the situation to our advantage.

"A team of psychologists ran an experiment where they planted women in a large psychology lecture," explained professor, *Platonic* author, and psychologist Dr. Marisa G. Franco. "The women were assigned to attend varying numbers of classes, ranging from none to most of them. At the end of the semester, [the researchers] asked the students in the lecture, 'Do you know who any of these women are?' And their answer was no, because it was a huge lecture. But they *also* asked them, 'How much do you like each of these women?' while showing the class pictures of the women, and they found that the women who showed up to the most classes were liked about twenty percent more than the women that didn't show up to any."[1] In their conscious minds, the other students didn't recognize *any* of the women. But somewhere in their subconscious brains, they'd decided they liked the people they were exposed to *more* than they liked the others simply because they were more familiar with their faces.

Dr. Franco explained that this was just one of many examples of the mere exposure effect, which is basically the idea that when people are familiar to us, we like them more. "They don't even have to say anything to us. It's completely unconscious," she said. "They also like *us* more."

One of the biggest mistakes we make when trying to make friends as adults is expecting friendships to form after a single exposure. I'm certainly guilty of this—I've expected friendship sparks to feel something like a platonic version of the love-at-first-sight referenced in movies. I want to find people I really *vibe* or *click* with. I'm disappointed when time spent with new potential friends doesn't feel as fun or effortless as time with people who are already in my life.

But *of course* it doesn't. I haven't allowed enough time for it to create that sense of ease. If you think about your current friendships, it creates an interesting chicken-or-egg cycle: Do we love our friends because we've spent so much time with them, and thus have "exposed" our way into affection, or do we spend so much time with our friends because we loved them in the first place?

Whichever it is, there's a definitive, actionable takeaway we can all use to take advantage of the mere exposure effect when we're trying to build new relationships, whether platonic or romantic, and that's to make recurring plans. If increasing exposure increases likability, the goal should be to make repeated exposure as streamlined as possible. Join a book club or a sports team or a language class. Have a weekly dinner party. Go to the same yoga studio for all your classes or the same café for all your lattes.

One of the best parts of the mere exposure effect is that it also gives you complete permission to feel a little weird or off initially, or like there's no "vibe" whatsoever—and, hopefully, the encouragement to persevere regardless. "Eventually, things are going to feel less awkward, and people are just going to be more likely to engage with one another," said Dr. Franco. "It's also helpful to keep in mind, because when I was in college, I showed up at one club event and no one really talked to me. I didn't connect with anyone, so my instinct was to not go back, even though it was after just one event. I didn't know that if I stayed for three months, if I actually committed, that's what was necessary to form those connections."

Figure out one recurring plan you can slot into your life. Because while there's obviously a certain ineffable quality to forming friendships, there's also a lot of very measurable science, and it's about time you used the data to your advantage.

51

Be a fun magnet.

We all know those people who just *feel good* to be around—*The Power of Fun* author Catherine Price calls them fun magnets, and it turns out anyone can become one. Price shared three steps to become the type of person who is both perceived as fun *and* attracts more fun into their life. (Don't worry—this process doesn't require being an extrovert in any way and is very much available to all of us.)

First, adopt the philosophy of "yes and," a practice derived from improv comedy. Price explained, "If someone has an idea that they put forth, and then the other person shoots it down, it kills the scene. Where are you supposed to go from there? Instead, you're supposed to say 'yes,' and then you're supposed to *build* on that idea"—that's the "and"—"so you're constantly providing new material for the scene. As many people in improv comedy have pointed out, it's a philosophy that can be applied to life as well."

The goal is to not immediately dismiss new ideas, but rather agree with or to them and build on them. "Try to notice your own impulse to respond with criticism or negativity, or even express self-criticism," said Price. "It might not immediately seem like you being self-deprecating will be a problem for other people, but actually, by criticizing yourself, you're encouraging other people to tune into that self-critic for themselves." Saying "I'm an awful bowler" might seem innocuous, but it invites anyone you're with to reflect on their own bowling skills. Are they a good bowler? And wait—do you need to be a *good* bowler to enjoy bowling? All of a sudden, a potentially fun evening has turned into a downer. What would it look like if instead, you tried bowling? If you put on the silly shoes and laughed at your gutter balls? If you agreed to go to the karaoke bar *and* suggested the group sing a song together?

The next step is to not put pressure on yourself to perform or be the funny one. Instead, *look for opportunities to laugh.* We often think the route to being fun or likable is being the star, telling captivating stories or having everyone bent over in stitches. In truth, we like people who make us feel good about *ourselves.* While someone who puts on a one-person show can be incredibly likable, it's much easier—and far more frequently successful—to be the person that makes others feel excited to share *their* stories and jokes.

I'll never forget a friend of mine who once described herself as being not particularly funny *but* quick to laugh. I happen to think she's funny, too, but the latter part is true: when I picture spending time with her, I see her full-body laughter, and it makes me immediately feel warm inside. I always feel amazing after we spend time together, and when she articulated her quick-to-laughness, I finally understood one of the reasons why. How refreshing is the notion that what people want to be around isn't necessarily the entertainer, but rather the person who is completely on board with being entertained? We spend so much time focusing on our jokes, but our laughter is one of the most beautiful gifts we can give people.

Last, Price suggested being intentional about giving people your full attention. Put your phone away, and truly listen to people when they talk. "People will really feel it, and they'll really appreciate it," said Price. "Regardless of whether or not fun ends up happening, the connection is going to be so much stronger."

Having tested Price's tips, though, I can say that fun—which she defines as "playful, connected flow"—will happen more often than not, and you'll experience the health and life benefits that come with it. Become a fun magnet, and watch the fun be drawn toward you.

52.

Practice habitual open-mindedness.

I first learned about the concept of habitual open-mindedness from famed psychologist and friendship expert Dr. Marisa G. Franco, and putting it into practice has changed how I interact with every single person in my life.

Habitual open-mindedness means approaching every interaction with every person you meet with no assumptions, no preconceived notions of who they might be. How a person looks or their place in society doesn't tell you anything about how they'll act, their behavior, or their character—you don't know anything about them. The goal is to allow each person to create themselves over time in front of you.

Dr. Franco shared an example from her own life of what it's like to be on the other side of a less open-minded interaction. "As a Black woman, people will be like, 'Hey, girl!' to me, and I'm like, 'You actually don't know how I talk.'"

Since speaking with Dr. Franco, every time I meet a new person, any time I catch myself making an assumption (negative *or* positive, the latter of which I actually find far more common): *I'm going to allow them to create who they are over time in front of me.* That simple sentence has opened me up to relationships with people of wildly different ages, political beliefs, backgrounds, and interests.

It also helps eliminate the sense of hierarchy, spoken or unspoken, that often limits the friendships we let ourselves form, even as we're telling ourselves that we want to level up the people we surround ourselves with. "Connection doesn't form well on a hierarchy," said Dr. Franco. "If you think people are better than you, it affects what we're willing to share with them. You don't want to be vulnerable with someone because you don't want them to judge you." When we're not being vulnerable, we're essentially sabotaging any connection we might have otherwise formed; not because we're on different social planes, but simply because time and again, research has shown that vulnerability facilitates connection (see page 179 for more on that).

If someone is wildly financially successful, let them create who they are over time in front of you. If someone is working three jobs to pay rent, let them create who they are over time in front of you. If someone is of any religion, identity, or social status: let them create who they are over time in front of you. We don't know who anyone is until they share themselves with us—when we assume who they are, we're not only likely to be wrong, we're putting obstacles in the path of a potential relationship.

53.

Become a winning
conversationalist.

I've been fairly vocal about hating small talk, and I don't think I'm alone in that. But I get it: it can be *hard* to know what to say to push the conversation past the weather, and soon enough, everyone is just standing there with "so . . ." eyes, looking for an exit opportunity. The secret, according to charisma expert and Science of People founder Vanessa Van Edwards, is to ask questions that we haven't answered over and over before, which snaps us out of autopilot.

"We did a huge speed-networking test where we assigned people different conversation starters and then had them rate their conversation in terms of quality," she explained. "We found that 'What do you do?' and 'How are you?' got the worst ratings. They created almost scripted, choppy conversations." Instead, in Van Edwards's research, these questions consistently got the best ratings:

"Working on anything exciting recently?"

"Have any fun or exciting plans coming up for the weekend?"

"What's been a recent big highlight for you?"

The goal is to create a question that's not *too* personal, so that it feels safe, but that differs from the norm and sets a positive tone (you're essentially prompting people to have excited thoughts, which they'll then associate with you). "Getting a little bit juicy with your willingness to ask slightly off-autopilot questions, that's what's going to get people really into talking to you," said Van Edwards. "It makes the conversation more memorable. It makes you more memorable."

But, I can hear you thinking, *what if the other person doesn't take the bait? What if they say, "No plans, really,"* or *"I haven't been working on anything fun"*? Well, according to Van Edwards, you have two options: "This is a courageous choice, but you can choose to put your conversational vulnerability out and answer first. You can say, 'Oh, well, no worries. I had a really slow week last week, too. This week, though, I'm super excited because I'm finally . . .'– fill in the blank," she explained. "You honor where they are—maybe even sharing a similar situation—and then you just go for it. Sometimes they just need a little bit of time to process. It's happened to me before where someone is so shocked by just not being asked 'What do you do?' that it took them two or three of my answers to realize they had something fun in their own life and then be willing to share it."

As for option two? It's a simple realization, but a powerful one: it's okay if not everyone is your person. "There are some people that you're just not going to click with," said Van Edwards. "And that's okay. That might not be your person." The good news is that you've lost *nothing* by putting yourself out there—who cares if you had a boring conversation with someone that's not going to impact your life meaningfully in the long (or even short!) run?

I also find it helpful to simply be vulnerable (see page 179) and admit that I hate small talk, and then either pull a card from one of the decks my conversation card company makes (yes, small talk annoys me so much that I started a company devoted to deep conversation—it's a perfect way to offload the vulnerability of the question onto the card) or say, "I heard a great conversation starter recently," and share a question I have at the ready. Eliminate the pressure to be naturally sparkly and witty and acknowledge instead that the vast majority of us are in the same boat—wanting to connect, wanting to talk about something *real* that lets us think and feel seen and heard, but finding that getting to that place isn't always easy or natural. You'll find that people are so relieved to not talk about the weather that it doesn't *matter* how you got there.

Finally, remember that one of the key elements of a top-tier conversation has nothing to do with talking: it's *listening*. Truly listening to what your conversational partner is saying will allow you to offer responses that are thoughtful, not rote, and will take the conversation down paths that are ultimately far more satisfying. We're often so worried about being witty or informed that we barely follow what the other person is saying, instead formulating our response while they talk. One of the biggest mistakes people make in conversation is thinking they need to be *interesting*. They'll share fun stories and jokes, and be exhausted by the end of the night from the pressure to perform.

When I spoke with Logan Ury, a top-tier dating coach, director of relationship science at the dating app Hinge, and author of the bestselling dating book *How to Not Die Alone*, she shared that the key to being liked by people, especially when you first meet them, is to be *interested*, not *interesting*. "Often, when I work with clients, they tell me they can't go out with anyone yet," she said. "They'll tell me they haven't gone on any cool trips recently, their job is boring, they have nothing to talk about. They're not *interesting* enough. They're so focused on how they're going to come across."

But, according to Ury, that's in contrast to the actual science of likability. "Research shows that asking people questions that make them feel interesting is what makes them attracted to you.[1] It's really about saying to someone, 'Oh, how did you end up moving here? How is this different from what you expected?'" she shared. "The more that the *other* person talks, the more they think that *you're* a great conversationalist."

While Ury's advice is focused on dating, it holds true for basically all human interactions. The next time you want someone to like you, ask them questions. You can ask them questions about topics that interest you, or even stick with more basic, universal questions. If you're struggling to figure out what to ask someone, psychologist Dr. Marisa G. Franco has a great tip that gets to the root of how people want to be listened to: look for the conversational cathexis. "This is a term psychologists use for where someone's emotional or intellectual energy is. What are they excited about?" said Dr. Franco. "For example, I was with a colleague, and we were talking about his son casually, and I noticed it was a cathexis for him—he lit up when he was talking about it. So I asked him, 'Have you always wanted to have kids? What's been your favorite part of fatherhood?'"

Ask better questions, and when people respond, be truly *interested*. Give other people the opportunity to shine, and don't be surprised when people suddenly think *you* light up the room.

54.

Deepen your existing friendships.

We all want to establish deep, intimate friendships, but sometimes, getting over the acquaintance hump can feel impossible. Even if we've created recurring plans and started to benefit from the intimacy formed from spending time together (see page 168), how do we get from there to late-night-phone-calls, share-all-our-secrets level? It turns out, the scientific community has figured out research-backed ways to create those deep relationships—and that having those deep social connections is critical for feeling good not only in our minds, but also in our bodies.

Dr. Robert Waldinger is the director of the Harvard Study of Adult Development, the longest study about human lives ever conducted,[1] and the author of the *New York Times* bestseller *The Good Life*. Over more than eighty years, researchers at Harvard followed the same individuals and their families, conducting thousands of surveys, doing brain scans and blood tests, and trying to get to the root of what makes people thrive. The answer it revealed is simple. "The single strongest predictor of thriving is good relationships with other people," Dr. Waldinger said when I interviewed him on one of my most downloaded podcast episodes ever. "It's not just emotional well-being and happiness—it's physical thriving. It's staying healthier longer and living longer."

Good relationships serve as stress-relievers. "Let's say that I have something really upsetting happen in my day, and I find myself ruminating about it," Dr. Waldinger explained. "I can feel my heart rate go up, and I can feel myself start to sweat. That's normal. Our bodies are meant to meet challenges by going into fight-or-flight response. But our bodies are also meant to return to baseline equilibrium when the threat goes away. If I come home and there's someone to talk to, or someone I can call, I can literally feel my body calm down. Good relationships regulate us. But if we don't have that person who we can talk to, scientific communities believe we stay in a chronic low-level fight-or-flight mode. We have higher levels of circulating stress hormones and levels of chronic inflammation."

This is where those research-backed ways to create deep relationships come in. In fact, according to friendship psychologist Dr. Marisa G. Franco, there's a three-step process to turn friends into closer friends or even best friends—and it's easier (and far more concrete and straightforward!) than you might imagine.

Step one: Decide whom you want to deepen your relationship with. "A lot of the time, we're really passive in our social worlds," said Dr. Franco. We hang out with the people who reach out to *us* instead of actively seeking out the type of people *we* want to hang out with (for more on that, see page 165). Bringing intentionality to your interactions is important for accessing subconscious levels of motivation, so choose a person with qualities you're actually looking to cultivate in your life. If you want to have a more fun-filled life, choose people who are quick to laugh and have a child-like sense of play. If you want to be pushed intellectually, choose someone who loves to learn and discuss. If you want someone to lounge around and watch reality TV with, well, choose someone who loves lounging and reality TV. It sounds simple, but if you're looking to have more adventures and you try to deepen a friendship with someone in a nesting phase, you'll not only disagree on how to spend time together, you'll feel a dissonance behind your interactions. Instead of serving as each other's expanders, you'll be limiting each other, which makes it hard to want to get close.

Step two: Get vulnerable. "We often think vulnerability burdens people," Dr. Franco said, "but according to the research, the more we intimately self-disclose, the more people like us."[2] Vulnerability can be sharing something you're embarrassed about. It can be announcing a dream you have, or disclosing a struggle you've been dealing with. It can also be saying, quite simply, "I've been wanting to fill my life with more meaningful friendships, and I really like you." Being vulnerable, at its core, is about being yourself, and trusting that other people will like you for that person, which is one reason Dr. Franco's research is so helpful—going into vulnerability knowing it *helps* people like you can make it less scary, and thus easier to simply show up as yourself. Being your truest self is a valuable long play. We're ultimately trying to find friendships that are the right fit for our unique selves, and the faster you can show that person, the quicker you can determine whether there's a match or lack thereof. Is the latter a bummer? Absolutely. But it's valuable information, and the sooner you have it, the sooner you can start deepening a friendship with someone who might be a better fit.

Step three: Show up for your friend in a time of need. "There are diagnostic moments in a friendship that disproportionately impact how we view it, and one is a moment when we really need support," said Dr. Franco. If a friend is sick, send them soup. If they're going through a hard time, send them a handwritten card, or call them and make sure they know you're available to talk.

If you're interested in deepening relationships in your life, think about step one, then look for opportunities for steps two and three. The resulting closeness you feel will make your efforts well worth it.

WANT TO DIVE DEEPER?

Listen to these episodes of **The Liz Moody Podcast:**

- "Tara Schuster—Practical Advice for Making Friends as an Adult, Career Success, Overcoming Depression and Anxiety & Forgiving Your Childhood," episode 45

- "Science-Backed Secrets for Making Friends as an Adult: Become Super Likable, Find Your BEST Friend, & Deepen Existing Relationships with Dr. Marisa G. Franco," episode 134
- "How to Have More Fun: Hidden Health Benefits, Becoming a Fun Magnet, & Phone Breakup Tips with Catherine Price," episode 133
- "How to Be More Attractive, Win at Apps, Flirt Better, and More: Relationship Scientist Logan Ury Answers YOUR Qs," episode 102
- "The Secret to Happiness, from the World's Longest Study with Dr. Robert Waldinger," episode 156

Explore these resources from our expert guests:

- *Buy Yourself the F*cking Lilies: And Other Rituals to Fix Your Life, from Someone Who's Been There* by Tara Schuster, @taraschuster on Instagram
- *Platonic: How the Science of Attachment Can Help You Make—and Keep—Friends* by Marisa G. Franco, PhD, www.DrMarisaG Franco.com
- *The Power of Fun: How to Feel Alive Again* by Catherine Price, www.ScreenLifeBalance.com
- *How to Not Die Alone: The Surprising Science That Will Help You Find Love* by Logan Ury, www.loganury.com
- *The Good Life: Lessons from the World's Longest Scientific Study of Happiness* by Dr. Robert Waldinger, www.robertwaldinger.com

HOW TO UPLEVEL YOUR LONG-TERM RELATIONSHIPS

55.

Be the CEO of your household.

Many of us say that we value our home life, yet we approach it with nowhere near the care, organization, or systemization that we give our work life—and then we wonder why it feels comparatively chaotic. Whether it's buying household goods or caring for children, our home lives are filled with hundreds of tasks that could benefit from care and optimization. And when we don't give them that attention, they can not only fall by the wayside but also create inequities in load distribution, which, in turn, can chip away at our individual energy and the integrity and intimacy of our relationships.

But what if we applied some of the managerial spirit from our workplaces to our home lives? Olivia Amitrano, who runs a thriving business, Organic Olivia, with her partner, Nick, shared her perspective with me: "You're the CEOs of your family." And part of being the CEO was establishing a routine of family meetings that has transformed her home life and relationship, a practice I've adopted with Zack and can enthusiastically vouch for.

Part one is the setup, where you figure out who owns which tasks and design an initial set of systems to keep those tasks humming along smoothly. Give yourself a good chunk of time to sit down, either by yourself, if you live alone, or with your partner or roommates. Write down all the tasks that are required to keep your household functioning, from the regular purchase of toilet paper to grocery shopping to home maintenance or childcare. Be as specific and realistic as possible—how often does grocery shopping need to happen? How often does the toilet paper need to be restocked? Then make sure there's a person assigned to each task—who may not be the person historically responsible for it. If you're in a partnership, this can be a helpful time to express any feelings about load inequities. It also serves to alleviate some of the more insidious elements of mental or emotional loads, where one person is responsible for keeping track of and assigning out household tasks, if not completing them, because you're sketching out the full task list and assigning the responsibility for each task together.

Once every task has been assigned, you're on to step two: designing systems to support each person in their tasks. Can anything be set up as an automated recurring order? Can you institute a plan for meals (Taco Tuesdays, Meal Prep Sundays) to eliminate decision fatigue around dinners each night? Can you set up autopay for your bills? If it's in the budget, you might also discuss outsourcing some tasks (see page 73).

Step three is the weekly meeting. Set a time that works for everyone involved to check in. I like to take a three-step approach to the meeting itself: First, we check in on everyone's designated tasks. Are certain things consistently falling by the wayside? What are some potential solutions? Have any new tasks cropped up that need to be assigned? Next, we look at our calendars for the upcoming week and sync up on any shared activities or events. This is also a great opportunity to ask for help when and if you need it: there have been weeks where I've been too busy to manage all my tasks, so we've made a plan for Zack to step in (and vice versa). One of the benefits of being in a partnership (or having roommates) is being able to help each other! This system is simply designed to keep one person from consistently taking on the bulk of the labor without appreciation or recognition, and to ensure all tasks are being completed by *someone* so the household runs as smoothly as possible. The last step that Zack and I add to the mix is a relationship check-in, where we ask each other the following questions:

- How did you feel cared for by me this week?
- What could I have done differently to care for you?
- How can I care for you in this coming week?
- What has been on your mind emotionally/practically/professionally this week? How can I support you in that?
- How can we include fun time/quality time/intimate time together this coming week?

The questions give us structure to check in with each other and make sure to nip any problems in the bud before they become larger resentments. I *love* our check-ins; they make me feel heard as a partner, and make me feel like I can show up better for Zack. They help give us back time and energy. They're both a signal we give to ourselves that our life outside work deserves the same thoughtful energy as our careers, *and* a way to eliminate unnecessary time sinks, stress factors, and dissonance.

56

Establish your rules for fighting.

According to John Kim, a licensed marriage and family therapist, bestselling author of *It's Not Me, It's You,* and podcast host, it's not inherently unhealthy to fight with your partner—the problem is in *how* we fight. Being able to truly understand your partner and having them seek to understand you is one of the most important elements of a relationship, and fighting—as uncomfortable as it might be in the moment—can be an important tool to get there.

The secret, according to Kim, is to establish the rules *before* you're in the weeds. "This is something that no one does. We just go into it," he said. "But you should definitely set rules, because otherwise, it isn't fair. It's like going into a fistfight with someone who has a gun."

A few of the rules Kim recommends are:

1. No character assassination. "You can't name-call someone or tell them they're generally awful," said Kim. "That's not going to go anywhere." Calling someone names or trying to break them down impedes what should be the ultimate goal of a fight: to work through the underlying difference of opinion or misunderstanding. You and your partner are on the same team, and

that team is only as strong as both of its players. Breaking down one player works against the team, and thus against your explicit interests. When I fight with Zack, I consciously remind myself of this to diffuse overpowering feelings of hurt and anger that crop up in the moment. We're fighting *for* our relationship, not *against* each other.

2. **No leaving without explicitly communicating it first.** "If you need a break, you have to tell the other person that you're coming back," Kim explained. A simple "I need to take a walk to clear my head, but I'll be back in fifteen minutes and ready to discuss this then" can go a long way in terms of creating space for clarity of thoughts while avoiding hurt feelings.

3. **Seek to understand before you seek to be understood.** "I used to go into conflict and conversations trying to prove a point, putting on my lawyer hat," said Kim. "I would try to get my partner to understand me first, instead of trying to understand her." He recommends flipping the situation and trying to understand your partner before you try to communicate your own point. This change transforms the dynamic of the conversation entirely. It shifts the focus from persuading to listening; instead of constructing your own rebuttal as your partner speaks, you're truly engaged in what they're saying. "It really creates a safe space," Kim said.

4. **Take ownership.** "This will look different for everyone," said Kim. "But there's an honesty to it. You're not just pointing fingers at your partner. Instead, you're holding up a mirror to yourself and saying, 'Here are *my* shortcomings. Here are *my* unhealthy patterns. Here's me putting old blueprints onto you.'" Treat it as a challenge—even if your gut instinct is that the onus is

on your partner, ask yourself what you might be con-
tributing to the situation, if you absolutely had to iden-
tify something. It's not absolving your partner of their
responsibility in the argument. Rather, it's acknowledg-
ing that every one of us is showing up to every moment
carrying all our past experiences. How we talk, feel, and
love is the culmination of our childhood, the lessons
we've internalized, what we've been rewarded and crit-
icized for. When two people interact, those past expe-
riences crash into each other both subtly and overtly.
Looking for how your past, present, and even future
have shaped the way you show up in the argument ac-
knowledges your understanding of that crash. It dif-
fuses the accusatory tension that often colors fights. It
says, *We're two people who've done the best we can with
what we've been given, and our goal in this moment is to
figure out how to do better together.*

Your fighting rules might look different, but it's worth consid-
ering what they are and, if you can, agreeing to them with your
partner. (If you can't agree, that's okay, too—at the end of the day,
we can only control ourselves, and simply establishing the rules
in your own mind will make a world of difference.)

PS: While Kim's therapy work is focused on couples in romantic
relationships, I've found his advice to be just as helpful when ap-
plied to other types of relationships, like those with family mem-
bers. Particularly, seeking to understand before being understood
has changed the dynamic of my conversations with my parents
and, as a result of that, how I approach difficult conversations in
general. Instead of something scary, they're opportunities to ex-
plore different perspectives. To grow. And, ultimately, to make my
relationships even stronger than they were before.

57.

Take your sex life to the next level.

If you want to take your sex life to the next level but have no idea where to begin, don't worry: Vanessa Marin has your back. Marin, a sex therapist and the author of *Sex Talks*, explained that the first place many of us want to start is with our confidence. "The first thing is to normalize *not* feeling confident," she said. "I've never met anybody who said, 'I'm one hundred percent wildly confident in the bedroom.' That just does not exist. All of us struggle in one way or another."

The thing with confidence, Marin shared, is that we let the abstract notion of not having it get in the way of having a great sex life, when really, we haven't even defined what that looks like in practice. "We fail to think about what that actually *means*," Marin said. "From a very practical standpoint, take the time to think about this question: What are the specific things that you would do if you had more confidence, or the specific ways that your sex life would be different if you had more confidence? 'I would try more sex positions.' 'I would get on top.' 'I would give my partner oral sex.' 'I would allow myself to receive oral sex.'"

These questions can point you in the direction of the sexual activities you'd like to integrate into your life. "We all want to be having great sex, but so few of us have taken the time to actually identify what that means to *us*," Marin said. "You can think about it more generally: What are the specific qualities or characteristics? You can even script out your ideal sexual experience from start to end. But sit with that question of, 'What is it that I'm even working towards in the first place?'"

Once you know *where* you want to go, the key to *getting* there is to take sexual baby steps. "We have this tendency to feel like it's all or nothing," Marin said. "But making little changes is actually going to feel so much more manageable, and it's going to keep that momentum going forward."

And when Marin said little changes, she meant *little*. "It could literally be something as small as 'I'm usually pretty quiet during sex, so I'm going to try breathing a little bit louder. Then maybe the *next* time I have sex, I'm going to try actually letting a few moans escape my mouth,'" she shared. "It's moving away from thinking you have to go from zero to sixty. It's taking tiny steps. Adjusting your position a little bit. Making a small request of your partner like, 'Can you kiss my neck?' If you normally have sex at night, could you try having morning sex? Or maybe afternoon sex?" (Interestingly, every sex or couples therapist I've had on the podcast has been a huge fan of scheduling sex. "It's such an underrated tool," said Marin. "We have this judgment of scheduling sex, but the reality is that most of us lead very scheduled lives, and we don't put judgment on the scheduling. We schedule date nights with each other. Do we ever judge that? No. We get excited about it." There's a lot of research to support that anticipating pleasure is enjoyable and contributes to our well-being,[1] which means that scheduling sex is only *adding* to the fun.)

Small changes like these not only allow us to have the positive experiences we need to keep moving forward in our sex lives, but they can also end up not being so small after all. "Small changes can actually make all the difference in the world," Marin said. "Sex positions are a great example. You can have the same sex position and put a pillow under your butt or change the placement of one of your limbs, and it actually feels like a totally different sex position. You don't need to research over-the-top poses or contort yourself." Licensed marriage and family therapist John Kim is a fan of adding a daily six-second kiss, a practice popularized by re-nowned psychologist Dr. John Gottman. "It breaks the pattern of us not being present with each other and connecting and just fall-ing into routines," Kim explained. "Whether we're talking about eating dinner, or making love, or watching TV, we all fall into these patterns where we're just on autopilot. And in that space, drift can happen. The six-second kiss breaks those patterns. Yes, it's weird. But the more awkward it is, the more telling it is that you should do it." Physical intimacy between partners also has well-researched benefits, including higher relationship satisfaction,[2] lower stress levels,[3] and increased levels of oxytocin (which leads to increased feelings of trust and closeness).[4]

Another small change is redefining what counts as "sex." Maybe one day, you take orgasms off the table. Maybe you play board games naked or meditate together or make out while you watch a movie. There are so many ways to be close, and leaning on all of them allows you to experience intimacy without the pressure that comes from a specific notion of bedroom activity with a race to the finish line.

If your tweaks don't go well the first time (or the first few times), know that you're not alone. In fact, the experience is so common, Marin and her husband, Xander, have a rule for it: the First Pan-cake Rule. "Some of our most bonding and intimate moments in the bedroom have been when we've tried something new and it went wrong. We didn't like the position, or someone farted in it, or we fell. But we can experience intimacy and connection regardless of how something goes," Marin explained. "When we make pan-cakes, the first one is just always kind of weird, and you don't know why. It's a way to lower expectations when you're trying something new—you can have this joke between the two of you, 'It's our first pancake. We're just tossing this one out. It's not going to count, but let's give ourselves permission to see how it goes.'"

At the end of the day, we're all just trying to feel the best we can. Pleasure isn't meant to be performative or perfect, and being sad-dled with those false expectations does nothing but hurt our sex-ual wellness. What does the sex life you want look like? And what's one tiny tweak you can make *today* to start that journey?

58.

Let your loved ones surprise you.

It's funny, isn't it, how we prioritize change and growth for ourselves, yet leave so little space for it in the people we love. I'm as guilty as anyone else of freezing friends, family members, and even my partner at a certain moment in time. I'll talk to Zack or my mom or dad or my best friend as if they're the version of themselves they were five years ago, while I'd be appalled if they did the same to me. What about all the work I've been doing? The books I've been reading, the trauma I've been tackling?

When I spoke with psychologist Dr. Samantha Boardman, she told me a story shared with her by her Harvard colleague, award-winning social psychologist Dr. Ellen Langer. "When couples would come to her after fifty years of marriage saying they wanted to divorce, there was often a common explanation," Dr. Boardman explained. "We think we can predict everything about our partners. 'Here they go again. They're going to do this and then they're going to watch TV and then they're going to shuffle to the kitchen and get a Coke,' and so on and so forth. When we assume people we love can't change, we limit their growth. Instead of reflecting their present self, the person they're likely trying to be, back at them, we're reflecting a person they've made efforts to evolve from."

The illusion of knowledge is damaging for both the person being perceived and the person doing the perceiving. On the part of the perceiver, it can make their partner feel incredibly unappealing: when we think we know how the story is going to end, we eliminate any reason to keep reading. And for the person being perceived, the perceptions are frequently limiting and often just plain wrong.

It's critical to regularly reflect on whether your relationship with your parents reflects who you all are today, versus your personalities and dynamics when you were growing up. Similarly, do you assume your partner will stick to behavior patterns established years, or even decades, ago? What about your friendships? Do you allow your friends to evolve in the same way that you have evolved during the time you've known each other?

Be your *most* curious self with the people you're closest to. Challenge yourself to look for something new when you interact with your loved ones. Let them write their story in real time, so every page turned boasts new opportunities for unexpected delight. You can even intentionally create space for people to surprise you: talk about topics that aren't normally part of your repertoire, or ask them to share something they've learned recently. Invite them to do an activity that you might have filed away as something they don't like. Maybe they enjoy it now! Or maybe they don't, but at least you've given them a new opportunity to share that information. You can even ask straightforwardly, "Is there any way you feel like you've grown or changed as a person that I might not be seeing or acknowledging?" It might be scary, but it might be an opportunity for a relational fresh start.

As a bonus, moving away from static conceptions of personality actually aids in our own growth. "We have these fixed ideas about ourselves and other people that dovetail with our longing to pursue certainty," Dr. Boardman said. "But our longing to be certain actually can distort our relationships with other people, and even our relationships to ourselves. There's something really beautiful about them being unknowable, and even ourselves being unknowable. There's something wonderful about being wrong and being surprised." I get it—I long for certainty, too. But there's a special, and even stronger, certainty that comes from giving people permission to be their most authentic selves with you. From letting people show you who they are rather than assuming you already know. From saying: "I trust that we can grow together."

WANT TO DIVE DEEPER?

Listen to these episodes of **The Liz Moody Podcast:**

- "Raw, Honest Tips for Upleveling Relationships: Get Your Needs Met, Ditch Toxic Patterns, & Amp Up the Passion with the Angry Therapist," episode 136
- "Herbalist Secrets for Better Periods, Sustained Energy, Healthy Hair, Lessened Anxiety & More with Organic Olivia," episode 130
- "How to Create Your Dream Sex Life, Have More Orgasms, Give Amazing Oral, & More with Vanessa and Xander Marin," episode 159

Explore these resources from our expert guests:

- *It's Not Me, It's You: Break the Blame Cycle. Relationship Better.* by John Kim, @theangrytherapist on social media
- Olivia Amitrano, @organic_olivia on Instagram
- *Sex Talks: The Five Conversations That Will Transform Your Love Life* by Vanessa Marin, vmtherapy.com

HOW TO
MAKE YOUR GUT
FEEL GREAT

59.

Eat thirty types of plants per week.

Every time I've interviewed a doctor, I've tried to ask them for the single best food to prioritize for health, and every time they've said the answer isn't a single food, it's as many *different* foods as possible—and plant-based foods, to be specific. While myopic focus on single "superfoods" is deemed by the media to be headline-worthy (remember the açaí craze? Or the kale era, or that time where coconut oil was apparently going to save our entire lives?), it's not the best way to approach eating well. In fact, a landmark international study called the American Gut Project found that the *number one* predictor of a healthy gut microbiome was diversity of plants in our diet.[1]

"Our microbiome is literally an ecosystem," explained renowned gastroenterologist Dr. Will Bulsiewicz. "Consuming a diverse array of plants is so important because every single plant has its own unique types of fiber." Microbes all have different dietary preferences—specific microbes like specific types of fiber and thus specific types of plants. The more plants you eat, the more types of microbes in your body will be fed and happy, and the more your microbiome will thrive, which will create downstream positive implications, from lessened inflammation[2] to better metabolic health.[3]

In the American Gut Project study, the number of different

plants consumed was thirty per week, which is the number that all of the doctors I interviewed suggested we aim for. "I know that sounds very overwhelming, but let me tell you how easy this can become," Dr. Bulsiewicz said. "Get whole wheat pasta and tomato sauce. Maybe we throw in some garlic and onions. Maybe we chop up some mushrooms, zucchini, maybe some spinach, then grab a handful of basil and add it to the sauce. You sit down to eat and then you throw some fresh parsley on top. Boom! Now you went from two up to like eight, nine, ten different plants without much effort. It tastes better, and your gut microbes are thriving."

Dr. Bulsiewicz suggests making the thirty plants per week a game, and even involving the whole family. "Kids love destroying their parents in a competition," he said. "Hang a sheet of paper on the fridge, write people's names, and start recording what plants they're eating, or how many different plants at each meal. I call them Plant Points. Every meal is an opportunity to score more Plant Points. This is a fun way to gamify this process."

Microbiome expert and author of *The Antiviral Gut* Dr. Robynne Chutkan likes what she calls her 1–2–3 rule: one plant at breakfast, two at lunch, and three at dinner. That way, you've had six plants by the end of the day, and you've hit thirty within five days.

Focusing on *adding* veggies to your meal is also a far more effective eating strategy than devoting your attention to what you're taking out. Deprivation-based diets don't work—studies have found that people who follow restrictive low-calorie diets often regain the weight, and these diets also increase stress[4] and the risk of developing disordered eating.[5] I can personally attest to all those things—in the years where I obsessively counted calories, not only did I develop an eating disorder, I also *still* spent every day hating my body. In fact, by viewing food in the context of numbers, I was constantly reinforcing the association that what I ate only mattered insofar as my weight and my body's physical appearance.

Switching to eating thirty plants per week will make a *huge* difference in your overall health, and that's without counting calories, eliminating food groups, or longing for a piece of pizza that you can't have (in fact, one of my all-time favorite easy weeknight meals is heating up a frozen pizza and making my go-to simple salad on the side—see the box on page 202!). You'll suddenly be eating more fiber, which will provide the prebiotic fuel your microbiome needs to thrive, and result in bowel movements you'll want to send text messages about. You'll be flooding your body with beneficial compounds that reduce inflammation[6] and risk of heart disease, stroke, type 2 diabetes, and certain types of cancer.[7]

Even cooler? You'll actually be altering your oral and gut microbiome in ways that make you crave *more* vegetables and less sugar.[8] Yes: the way you become a person who loves nutrient-dense food is by eating nutrient-dense food, kick-starting a positive feedback cycle that happens on both a physiological and a psychological level. And best of all? All this works together to underscore a different association: that your body is for *living*, not looking. Every action you take is a powerful vote toward *your* experience of *your* body. When you're eating to try to make it appear a certain way? That's telling your brain that your body is for looking. When you're eating to make it *feel* a certain way? That's telling your brain that your body is just the tool through which you get to *live*.

I'm gonna be honest with you: even I don't metabolically optimize every meal I consume, or make sure every bite I take is as nutrient-dense as possible (see page 226). What I *do* do, for almost every meal, almost every day, is find a way to add at least one plant, my own simplified way of pushing toward the thirty-plants-per-week goal. And if I can't add it in a seamless, delicious way (which is always my preference—I've shared ideas to get you started here!), I simply grab a carrot, celery, or other crudités-tray-worthy vegetable and munch it along with whatever I'm eating. I order a veggie side off the menu. I make the world's fastest salad by simply drizzling olive oil and sprinkling salt on whatever greens I have on hand.

Ditch restriction and aim to eat thirty plants a week. It'll make your food more delicious, it'll transform your health, it'll change your view of the role of food in your life, and, bite by bite, I promise, it'll change your life.

MY FAVORITE WAYS TO ADD MORE VEGGIES TO YOUR DAY

Breakfast:

- Make a green smoothie.

- Wilt spinach into your scrambled eggs.

- Make individual veggie frittatas in a muffin tin, then store in the freezer to grab and go.

- Add some mashed sweet potato to your oatmeal.

- Crumble some crispy kale chips on top of your avocado toast.

- Make a pesto sauce and fry or scramble an egg in it.

- Make a breakfast salad with a fried egg on top.

- Make a Brussels sprout–based hash, then freeze it on sheet pans (to prevent clumping) before transferring to a large freezer-safe container from which you can dole out individual servings.

Lunch

- Add lettuce or fresh herbs to your sandwich.

- Sauté some kale for a quick quesadilla (I like to do cheese, sautéed kale, some salt, onion powder, and garlic powder between two tortillas of choice—it takes ten minutes and is incredibly crave-worthy!).

- Meal prep a salad or soup that you can stash in jars in your fridge to grab and go all week.

- Add onions and peppers to your burrito bowl order.

- Blend cooked zucchini, carrots, cauliflower, peppers, or any other veggies into pasta sauce for added nutrients you won't even notice.

Dinner

- Swap out half your white rice for cauliflower rice (it actually adds a beautiful nutty flavor to dishes but is *far* more satisfying when mixed with regular rice).

- Swap out half your ground beef for finely chopped mushrooms.

- Make a side salad for a frozen pizza (I make my go-to dressing by zesting a lemon and grating garlic directly onto lightly salted greens using a Microplane—one of my favorite affordable kitchen tools—then squeeze on the lemon juice and finish with a bit of olive oil—it's simple but so satisfying).

- Graze on carrots and hummus while you cook.

- Roast frozen cauliflower or broccoli to serve as a side dish to any meal. (My trick: Roast it on a parchment paper–lined pan at 400°F with no oil or seasonings until it's brown at the edges, 25 to 30 minutes—this lets the moisture evaporate. Then toss with a drizzle of oil, salt, and whatever seasonings you'd like and return to the oven for 7 to 10 minutes more, until brown and crispy. I always keep bags of broccoli and cauliflower in my freezer so I can use this method to add a veggie to any meal that needs it!)

- Top any meal with fresh herbs.

60.

Cook and cool your carbs.

There's not much I love more than taking a good meal I'm already eating and making it even better for me by doing—well, nothing. Allow me to introduce you to the concept of resistant starches, which always feels like nature performing a magic trick. Essentially, if you cook certain simple starches like pasta or rice and then let them cool, they *change molecular structure* and become what are called resistant starches.

World-renowned gastroenterologist Dr. Robynne Chutkan explained: "Resistant starches are a specific type of carbohydrate that aren't broken down in your small intestine, which is where carbohydrate digestion generally happens. Instead, they travel through your GI tract relatively intact until they reach your colon, where they're fermented by gut bacteria to produce important substances called short-chain fatty acids, or SCFAs. SCFAs like butyrate are extremely important for colonic health: they're a primary energy source for colonic cells, they have anti-inflammatory and anticarcinogenic properties,[1] and they've been shown to increase absorption of minerals."[2] SFCAs can stimulate the release of insulin and improve the glucose absorption of muscles,[3] which helps mitigate the blood sugar roller coaster many of us experience after eating a carb-heavy meal.[4] They also digest more slowly, which helps further mitigate that blood sugar response. (For more on the many health benefits of SCFAs, see page 214.)

"Resistant starches function more like dietary fiber than starch,

encouraging the growth of healthy microbes in the colon and act-
ing as a prebiotic food, one that actually feeds gut bacteria and re-
duces production of potentially harmful compounds such as bile
acids and ammonia," explained Dr. Chutkan.[5]

There are a few ways to increase the amount of resistant starch
in your diet. The first is to eat more type 2 resistant starch, which
is found naturally in unripe bananas (as they ripen, going from
green to yellow, the starches turn into sugars), oats, and cashews.
This type of resistant starch actually decreases when you cook the
food, so if, for instance, you like cooked oatmeal and overnight
oats equally as much, choosing the latter would provide more re-
sistant starches.

The second way, and my absolute favorite, is to cook and cool
certain foods, like potatoes, rice, pasta, legumes, and corn, which
creates type 3 resistant starches (this is also called starch retrogra-
dation).[6] Simply cook them as usual, then let them cool down com-
pletely, which causes the amylose and amylopectin molecules in
the starch to re-form into a more crystalline structure that is more
resistant to digestion (as a person who's terrified of food poison-
ing, I'd be remiss to not take this opportunity to remind you that
rice and some other grains often contain a bacteria called *Bacillus
cereus* that can cause gastrointestinal distress when not handled
properly; because of this, you want to get them into the fridge as
quickly as possible after cooking if you're not eating right away,
and *never* leave them sitting out on the countertop for an extended
period of time).

Even cooler? The majority of that resistant starch *stays present*
even after the food in question is reheated. Yes, that means you can
roast a sweet potato for dinner tonight, eat some, store the rest in
the fridge, and then reheat it the very next night—and with zero ef-
fort on your part, it'll suddenly be even better for your blood sugar
and your gut. A number of things impact the amount of type 3
resistant starch in a food, including how long it's cooled for (in
general, 24 hours in the fridge creates more resistant starch than
quickly cooling to room temperature), the cooking method, and
the amounts of various types of starch in the food in the first place.

But in general, I view this tip as an excellent opportunity to embrace leftovers, which I think are not nearly as lauded as they should be. The only thing better than having a little gift from past you in the fridge, ready and waiting to satiate you when hunger strikes, is knowing that that gift is going to serve as fuel for your gut, even though you've done nothing different to it. When you make a pasta dinner, make a few servings and eat some for lunch the next day. Roast some sweet potatoes at the beginning of the week and store them in the fridge so they're ready to eat with some olive oil, salt, and cinnamon when hunger strikes. Make a potato salad for your next potluck. Your gut will thank you.

61.

Incorporate more fermented foods.

When three separate world-class doctors bring up the same study in different conversations, you pay attention. The study in question, conducted by the Stanford University School of Medicine, was explained to me by top gastroenterologist Dr. Will Bulsiewicz. "When people added fermented foods to their diet, they were able to enhance the health of their gut microbiome in ten weeks,"[1] he shared. In addition, immune cells showed less activation in the group that ate fermented food, and nineteen inflammatory proteins measured in blood samples also decreased.[2]

"The microbes in fermented food bring out the best of it. They create new vitamins. They create new forms of fiber. They transform the polyphenols," Dr. Bulsiewicz said. Metabolic health expert Dr. Casey Means cited fermented foods as one of the core components of a metabolically healthy plate (see page 49), and doctor after doctor shared how they personally try to fill their diets with as many fermented foods as possible. In fact, outside of vegetables, fermented foods were *the number one* thing that experts on the podcast most often recommended adding to our plates.

Fermented food is one of the single best dietary additions to decrease inflammation,[3] which is at the root of many health conditions, and increase the health of the microbiome, which, via the trillions of bacteria that populate every part of us, impacts the health of the whole body. I've also found it immensely helpful with my own sugar cravings, which could be explained in part because of the positive effect on our gut or oral microbiome (as the microbes shift, so too do our cravings!), metabolic health (when your blood sugar isn't spiking and crashing, you crave less food that *makes* it spike and crash), and/or inflammation levels. It could also simply be due to their funky sour taste, which almost feels like a palate reset. However it works, fermented foods have become one of my favorite ways to avoid sweets when I'm eating them mindlessly versus truly savoring them: I'll eat a spoonful of fermented carrots or sauerkraut on its own, and instantly my craving goes away.

The variety of fermented foods available today has never been wider, and they're fun and tasty to experiment with in your cooking. Pick up some fermented salsa or hot sauce (I usually find some at my local farmers' market, or you can make your own!) and add it to eggs, stir-fries, and tacos. Grab some fermented beets, carrots, or sauerkraut and add a spoonful to salads or roasted meats or veggies. Make a bowl of miso soup or take a swig from a bottle of kefir.

Beyond the health benefits and craving conquering ability, it just makes food taste better, adding depth, complexity, and interest to meals. Aim to add fermented food to one meal a day, and increase the number from there.

62.

Get dirty.

If you ever go on a hike with me, you'll see me stop and occasionally rest my hands on boulders. It's a weird habit that I've had for as long as I can remember: as my dad was dragging me up the seventh mile of our "quick, easy stroll," I always felt like the large rocks infused me with the extra power that I desperately needed.

While rocks might not actually infuse us with energy, it turns out, they do have some healing powers. The acts of simply touching nature, and getting your skin a little dirty, or leaving a little dirt on your food, are actually one of the best ways to take care of your microbiome. Renowned Yale-trained dermatologist and *The Beauty of Dirty Skin* author Dr. Whitney Bowe explained: "Healthy skin is not squeaky-clean skin. Our obsession with this 'squeaky-clean' feeling and our antiseptic hygiene habits are disrupting and destroying the health of our skin's barrier."

The skin microbiome is just one of many microbiomes in the body, including our skin oral microbiome, nasal microbiome, genital microbiome, and, of course, our famous gut microbiome, and for all of them, chasing that squeaky-clean feeling often means wiping out the diversity and quantity of bacteria living within them. This is one of many reasons that every doctor I've ever interviewed recommends against intravaginal cleansing, or douching, and colonics, which, despite being incredibly trendy in the wellness world at times, can have destructive effects on the gut microbiome (if you're constipated, see page 217 for more microbiome-friendly ways of getting things moving).

Because of that microbiome effect, getting dirty can be beneficial for many aspects of our health. In an effort to figure out the skyrocketing rates of autoimmune phenomena in British children, Dr. David Strachan, an epidemiologist at the Royal School of Tropical Medicine and Hygiene, embarked on a twenty-one-year study following 17,000 children from birth to adulthood. His results, published in 1989, found two startling factors.[1]

"The first," explained gastroenterologist Dr. Robynne Chutkan when we spoke on my podcast, "was that kids from large families where somebody was always sick—a brother or a sister or cousin always had the flu, or cough, or cold—were much less likely to have autoimmune diseases later on. Essentially, their immune system was being trained not to overreact later. The second finding was even more unexpected: kids from households where there was more general sanitation had higher rates of autoimmune disease later in life."

Dr. Strachan's discovery turned our entire notion of cleanliness on its head, and highlighted the necessity of maintaining the health of our microbiomes in order to maintain protection against chronic diseases. To be completely clear, this doesn't go against Louis Pasteur's germ theory: we still want to do our best to avoid the pathogenic bacteria, viruses, and fungi that can cause *acute* sickness. But we also want to do our best to avoid autoimmune reactions that lead to *chronic* sickness, which involves protecting our microbiomes when possible, and certainly avoiding needlessly destroying them. We're just at the beginning of our research into the microbiome, and we're learning more every single year about just how important having a healthy microbiome is to our oral health, gut health, skin health, and more.

This book is stacked with tips for helping our various microbiomes thrive (see pages 199, 204, 207, and 214), but one of my favorites is simply to lean into nature, both in terms of the food we eat and what we expose our skin to. "Pets in the household can increase the diversity of bacteria and can be beneficial for our immune development," shared Dr. Bowe. "Travel to rural environments and spend time in nature. Scientists who have traveled to rural locations and sampled their own skin and gut every day have seen beneficial changes within a matter of days."

Some other tips? Avoid oversanitizing your home, and you don't need the antibacterial handwash: the FDA has acknowledged that normal soap and water is just as effective and kills far less of the good bacteria on your skin. There's also a lot of research around the health benefits of gardening, which range from reduced stress to a more diverse gut microbiome[2] to reduced risk of heart attack and cardiovascular disease.[3] While there are a variety of factors at play, one of them is the act of engaging with the robust microbiome of the soil—that is, getting your hands dirty.

I also personally use this tip to justify my love of rock-touching, but also as simply another motivating reason to get in nature: to sit on grass, go for hikes, and generally get dirty in a way that our society rarely encourages. (Do I also use it to sometimes justify my personal messiness at home? Maybe. Sorry, Zack.) Since interviewing Dr. Bowe, I now also think about my skincare in terms of my skin microbiome and skin barrier versus trying to get it as clean as possible. "When we overscrub and overexfoliate our skin, we are compromising our skin's delicate barrier, which gives rise to sensitive, irritated skin, not optimized, healthy, nourished skin," she explained.

We're not shiny pieces of plastic—we're living, breathing collections of trillions of bacteria, and we need to cultivate an environment for them to thrive.

63.

Don't unnecessarily
eliminate foods.

I'm a huge advocate of taking an additive approach to health—how can we fill our diets and days with a diversity of foods and activities and interactions that fuel and satiate us? Diet culture can often masquerade as health culture, with soft promises of bellies made flat by the removal of entire food groups. Yet most foods, consumed in moderation, aren't a problem for most people, and the demonization of so many foods is making people approach dining with fear rather than joy (which can actually lead to cascading negative effects that the removal of the foods was meant to solve, since stress can cause inflammation that can lead to gastrointestinal distress,[1] among other things). That's why I was so happy when renowned gastroenterologist Dr. Will Bulsiewicz shared his philosophy for healthy eating, which centers on celebrating the beneficial properties of food.

Dr. Bulsiewicz rarely suggests people avoid entire food groups. "The gut is like a muscle. It can be trained. It can be strengthened. But if you stop using it, it will grow weaker," he explained. "Let's pretend that you're sensitive to beans. Just like with exercise, there is a certain threshold that you are capable of. If I go to the gym and I lift three times my normal amount, I'm going to hurt myself. Don't go for the four-bean chili if you're not used to eating beans, or if beans cause trouble. But there is a threshold, where if you stay below that threshold and you introduce beans in the right amount of moderation, just like with exercise, the right amount of exercise puts the right amount of stress on your body. We call it eustress. The right amount of stress is healthy stress, and it makes you stronger. Take it super slow and recognize that just like with exercise, there might be some discomfort."

Rather than eliminating certain foods for the rest of their lives, Dr. Bulsiewicz prefers to have patients focus on strengthening their gut. "I worry about the idea that if it hurts your gut, you should eliminate it. That, to me, is the biggest misconception," he said. "Studies show that when people eliminate foods from their diet, they end up with a less healthy gut.[2] I see these people in my clinic, and they say they felt better for a few weeks, but now they're worse than when they started. They get on a progressively more restricted diet to address the worsening symptoms because they believe that this is what they're supposed to do to heal their gut. The next thing you know, all they're eating is boiled chicken and potatoes."

While some people will need to eliminate full categories of food (no amount of gut strengthening will make gluten a good choice for someone with celiac disease), far too many of us are limiting what we put on our plate in ways that are making our gut health worse—not better. Dr. Will suggests that instead of unnecessarily eliminating foods, we focus on strengthening the health of our gut so that it can absorb and digest as wide of a range of foods as possible (see pages 199, 207, and 214). If you are experiencing gastrointestinal distress, consider consulting with a registered dietitian or gastroenterologist. Experiment with eating smaller amounts of certain foods or food groups until you find your own personal balance. But don't categorically get rid of foods without a very good reason—it's worse for your gut *and* your quality of life.

64.

Feed your good gut bacteria.

You've likely heard of probiotics, the good bacteria that populate our microbiomes, and maybe you've even heard of prebiotics, the food those bacteria need to thrive. But have you heard of postbiotics? These are the by-products of the fermentation process carried out by the probiotics; essentially, when the probiotics *digest* the prebiotics, they produce postbiotics. And those postbiotics are a critical element for maintaining a healthy gut,[1] which in turn impacts the health of our whole bodies.

Short-chain fatty acids (SCFAs) are one of the most well-researched types of postbiotics. "Short-chain fatty acids like acetate, butyrate, and propionate are essential for maintaining a healthy gut lining," explained board-certified integrative gastroenterologist Dr. Robynne Chutkan. There are also studies that point to the anti-inflammatory, antitumor, and antimicrobial effects of SCFAs,[2] making optimizing your SCFA production a worthy goal for a host of desired outcomes.

"Studies have shown that people who responded well to cancer therapy had higher numbers of the butyrate, or short-chain fatty acid–producing microbes,"[3] shared gastroenterologist Dr. Will Bulsiewicz. The key to producing SCFAs is to consume plant fiber (the prebiotic), which will be fermented by the probiotics in your microbiome into SCFAs (the postbiotic).

"In the study, if you ate at least twenty grams of fiber per day, you were more likely to survive and be free of melanoma with immunotherapy,"[4] shared Dr. Bulsiewicz. "Every five grams of fiber led to a *thirty percent increased likelihood of survival*. It parallels colon cancer research, where they've looked at diet after a person is diagnosed with colon cancer. They found that every five grams of fiber people added to their diet increased their likelihood of survival by eighteen percent."[5]

While all plant fibers are correlated with postbiotic production, one of the largest producers of SCFAs, and particularly butyrate, is a bacteria called *Faecalibacterium prausnitzii*, or *F. prausnitzii*. "That type of bacteria is most likely to ferment when fed a type of fiber called inulin, which is the dense, stringy fiber found in foods like artichokes, asparagus, garlic, leeks, and onions," explained Dr. Chutkan.

One of Dr. Chutkan's favorite SCFA-producing recipes is a soup that's her go-to when she's feeling sick and wants to have that extra infusion of microbiome support. If you'd like to try it yourself (it's become a regular for microbiome support in my house, and I know many of you have sworn by it), I've included the recipe here. Enjoy!

DR. CHUTKAN'S SHORT-CHAIN FATTY ACID SUPPORTIVE SOUP

Makes 1 large serving

2 leeks
Olive oil
1 yellow onion, coarsely chopped
1 jalapeño, stemmed, seeded, and coarsely chopped
Fine grain sea salt
½ cup canned coconut milk (lite and full-fat both work!)
1 cup veggie broth
3 green onions, coarsely chopped
3 garlic cloves, coarsely chopped
Juice of 1 lime
½ teaspoon curry powder
½ teaspoon ground turmeric

Slice off the root ends and woody tops of the leeks and cut the leeks in half lengthwise. Rinse well to remove any grit between their layers, then coarsely chop them.

In a medium pot, warm a drizzle of olive oil over medium heat. Add the onion, leeks, jalapeño, and a pinch of salt. Cook, stirring regularly, until just golden. Add the coconut milk, broth, green onions, and garlic. Bring the mixture just to a boil, then remove from the heat. Add the lime juice, curry powder, and turmeric. Carefully transfer to a standing blender or blend directly in the pot with an immersion blender until smooth. Taste and season with additional salt, if desired. Enjoy!

65.

Eliminate bloating
and constipation.

You might not think of pooping as a critical wellness practice. If that's the case—well, you're sorely mistaken. Regular bowel movements are vitally important to our overall health. "Research has clearly shown that the appearance of our bowel movements and the amount of time food spends in our intestines (referred to as transit time) are associated with specific patterns in our gut microbiome,"[1] reported gastroenterologist Dr. Will Bulsiewicz. "Given the connections of our gut microbiome to so many aspects of human health including digestion, our metabolism, our mental health, our hormones, and our immune system, this speaks to the importance of maintaining regular, healthy, complete bowel movements. More simply put, don't you feel awesome when you have a fantastic bowel movement? Yeah, me too. There's a reason for that."

If you're bloated, one of the main culprits might be—you guessed it—not pooping enough. In fact, according to Dr. Bulsiewicz, it's the number one cause of bloating. "The people who are like, 'Hey, I woke up and my stomach looked normal, and then a couple hours later it's completely distended,' it's almost always constipation, and they may not realize it," he said. "They may be pooping every day and may not realize that they're still constipated because they're not completely emptying."

The first step to becoming an A+ pooper is simply recognizing pooping's place as a critically important tool in your wellness arsenal. Don't worry—after that, we have some key practical strategies you can employ as well.

One tip is to recognize that your microbiome, like most of the rest of your body, runs on your circadian clock. Because of this, it's important to create and stick to a pooping routine as much as possible. "You can train yourself to poop at the same time every day. It's like potty training a child—if you sit on the toilet at the same time every day, you will form a habit," said Dr. Bulsiewicz. "Once a day, at the time that you want to build the habit, sit on the toilet for five minutes. Don't strain. Don't push. Don't force it. If five minutes go by and you don't go, just leave. But if you do this at the same time every day, your body will actually pick up on what you're trying to do."

Paying attention to the physical position of your body can help with evacuation as well. "Throughout human history prior to very recently, we pooped in a squatted position. There's actually a muscle called the puborectalis that's like a sling muscle that doesn't fully straighten out your rectum unless you're in a squatted position," Dr. Bulsiewicz explained. "You can purchase a Squatty Potty, or you can just have a box or a stool that you put your feet up on. The important point is to have your knees above your hips."

Physical movement, hydration, and consuming enough fiber (especially in conjunction with hydration—too much fiber without enough water can actually have the opposite of the intended effect) were also top doctor recommendations for pooping. While everybody is different, aiming for one bowel movement a day is a good ballpark to meet typical health needs.

Dr. Bulsiewicz also suggests using magnesium to help evacuate the bowels. "Magnesium glycinate is absorbed more easily, so when you want the magnesium in your blood for things like anxiety or migraines, that should be your go-to," he said. "To get a bowel movement, you need to actually overwhelm your gut's ability to absorb the magnesium by taking a certain amount of it all at once to draw water into the colon and then flush through." For that, he recommends magnesium citrate, starting with 250mg and going up to as much as 500mg at a time. This should be done under the direction of a healthcare provider, who can check your magnesium levels before and after initiating the magnesium and also make sure it's a good choice within the context of your personal medical history.

If all of the above doesn't work, and *especially* if it doesn't work and you've given birth, Dr. Bulsiewicz recommends looking into pelvic floor therapy. "If a person has a pelvic floor dysfunction, then you can do everything right and still not poop. If you can't open the bottom, then it doesn't matter what the motility is. You're running into a brick wall. This is the person who strains to have a bowel movement even when it's a soft bowel movement. This is the person who goes and feels like they don't completely go. This is the person who has little nuggets for bowel movements, not logs. The person who poops once, and then has to poop again thirty minutes later. These are all suggestions of the possibility of pelvic dysfunction."

Explore the various constipation-relieving options and see what works for you—and if none do, it's worth talking to a pelvic floor specialist or a gastroenterologist about pelvic floor dysfunction. The key takeaway? Consider pooping a critical part of your daily health routine, as important (if not more so!) as the more traditionally talked about parts of wellness.

WANT TO DIVE DEEPER?

Listen to these episodes of The Liz Moody Podcast:

- "The Future of Gut Health: Cancer Treatment, Circadian Rhythms, Mental Health Advancements, and So Much More with Dr. Will Bulsiewicz," episode 113
- "Ask the Doctor: Gut Health Edition—Eliminating Bloat & Constipation, the Best Supplements, Nourishing Your Microbiome and MUCH More with Will Bulsiewicz, MD," episode 43

- "Gut Health Secrets: The Truth About Leaky Gut, Viral Infections, Chronic Disease & Acid Reflux with Dr. Robynne Chutkan," episode 142
- "Ask the Doctor: Debunking Skin Care Myths—Slugging, Face Shaving, Red Light, Collagen, Ice Rollers & More with Dr. Whitney Bowe," episode 127

Explore these resources from our expert guests:

- *Fiber Fueled: The Plant-Based Gut Health Program for Losing Weight, Restoring Your Health, and Optimizing Your Microbiome* by Will Bulsiewicz, @theguthealthmd on Instagram and Facebook, @theguthealthmd_ on TikTok
- *The Anti-Viral Gut: Tackling Pathogens from the Inside Out* by Dr. Robynne Chutkan, www.RobynneChutkan.com
- *The Beauty of Dirty Skin: The Surprising Science of Looking and Feeling Radiant from the Inside Out* by Dr. Whitney Bowe, @drwhitneybowe on Instagram

HOW TO
LIVE LONGER

66.

Reframe stress relief.

We all know that stress is bad for our health, but the concept of "stress reduction" can feel vague, and often falls to the bottom of our priority list. I get thousands of messages from people who are trying to perfect the last 5 percent of their diet or supplement routine while running around frazzled from the moment they wake up until the moment their head hits the pillow—and even causing *more* stress in the pursuit of a notion of "perfect wellness."

If that sounds like you, you might need to hear this: As it turns out, chronic stress is associated with increased levels of inflammation.[1] And chronic inflammation is at the root of pretty much every disease.

Dr. Heather Moday, integrative immunologist and author of *The Immunotype Breakthrough*, broke it down like this: "Inflammation is part of what our immune system does. If we didn't have an active immune system, we would die. When we injure ourselves, there are certain immune cells that come to the area and shoot off flares in the form of chemicals—usually cytokines. They cause blood vessels to dilate, which brings more fluid to the area and causes heat and swelling. If there's a bacterial infection and viral infection, those cytokines start to do a lot of the killing. This sometimes creates some collateral damage to the tissue around it that then has to be cleaned up."[2] Dr. Moday likens the experience to a forest fire—you end up putting out the fire or taking care of the inflammation, but there's damage to the area as you do that. That unintentional damage, according to Dr. Moday, is one of the paths to chronic in-flammation.

The other cause of chronic inflammation, though, is constant, prolonged exposure to something causing an inflammatory re-sponse. "If you never get rid of the initial cause of the inflamma-tion, it's like keeping that fire constantly smoldering," Dr. Moday explained. That source could be something like pollution, foods, cigarette smoke, alcohol—or, notably, stress. "Stress acts in a bell curve," explained Dr. Moday. "Acute intermittent stress is actually anti-inflammatory because cortisol acts on receptors on immune cells to reduce the expression of cytokines [this is the concept of hormesis, explained on page 64]. In long-term stress, the theory is that the cortisol receptors on cells become less responsive or even resistant to the turning off of these cytokines." This causes a vicious cycle where you continue to become inflamed, which recruits those cytokines, which creates more collateral damage, which causes more inflammation.

All that chronic inflammation can create various states of dis-comfort in our bodies. "Over time, cortisol has been shown to cause ongoing tissue damage in several organs—notably, the brain," ex-plained Dr. Moday. "It's been associated with actual structural changes in the brain, as well as depression.[3] Because of the in-creased tissue damage due to that cortisol resistance, there are links to autoimmune disease[4] and cardiovascular disease[5] as well. With chronic GI issues like cramping or bloating, there's usually some inflammation going on. Joint pain is a big symptom of in-flammation. Chronic hives or other skin conditions can be indica-tive of chronic inflammation, as can having your brain feel slow or sluggish.[6] Chronic stress can downregulate the activity of cancer-seeking killer T cells and NK cells, which is one of the reasons it has been implicated as a risk factor for malignancy.[7]

The good news? "There are a lot of things that we can do to try to reregulate our autonomic nervous system and our adrenals, because we do know that that also significantly impacts how our inflammation levels and immune system work," said Dr. Moday. There are plenty of practices to experiment with (including many in this book; see pages 154, 249, and 254); Dr. Moday personally loves gratitude journaling, time in nature, and deep-breathing exercises. The key, though, is to realize stress isn't some esoteric thing that at most will make your day feel a little worse. Stress actually has concrete physiological effects and real health consequences. It's as important to prioritize stress reduction as it is to move your body and eat well, yet often we treat it like something we can put off for a future time, or the earned result of going through *enough* stress, finally accomplishing *enough*.

Stress is hurting your body *now*. Reframe stress reduction to be a nonnegotiable health priority. Doctor's orders.

67.

Maximize the amount of nutrients per bite.

A huge percentage of the U.S. population isn't getting enough of key vitamins and minerals: 94 percent of people don't get enough vitamin D, 88 percent don't get enough vitamin E, 52 percent don't get enough magnesium, 44 percent don't get enough calcium, 43 percent don't get enough vitamin A, and 38 percent don't get enough vitamin C. Most people aren't getting enough potassium, choline, vitamin K, B vitamins, copper, selenium, and zinc.[1] And this is a problem, because these micronutrients (and many others) play a hugely important role in our overall health. "We talk a lot about macronutrients—fat, protein, carbs," said Stanford-trained metabolic health expert Dr. Casey Means. "But the little molecules that actually make the cell work properly are the micronutrients." Dr. Means explained that the energy that fuels all our cells, known as adenosine triphosphate (ATP), can only be created if we have sufficient micronutrients to do so. When we're deficient in ATP, we're like cars without enough fuel. It doesn't matter what else you do to the car—if you get cool hubcaps or new tires—without fuel, you can't turn on the engine. Without ATP, our cells are essentially stuck, useless, sitting in the driveway.

Micronutrient deficiency comes down to two main factors, said Dr. Means. The first is the health of the soil in which our food is grown—if the soil itself is depleted of biodiversity, the plants it produces will be less nutrient-rich, which negatively impacts our bodies when we consume these plants as food. Unfortunately, studies show that the concentration of nutrients in our food has drastically decreased in the last few decades. This could be due to a variety of reasons, such as intensive agriculture, pesticide use, deforestation, habitat fragmentation, climate change, and plastic pollution.[2]

"Even if you're eating a rich diversity of unprocessed plant foods, the food now just has much less nutrient value," Dr. Means explained. "Even in meat, animal protein from animals raised on regenerative soil has more micronutrients, healthy fats, and phytonutrients—but those animals have to be eating nutrient- and phytonutrient-rich plants.[3] It's a whole cycle." Step one, then, would be an awareness of the connectivity of how we treat our land and the resulting outcomes in our body, and advocating and voting for systemic changes.

Step two, though, is actionable at this very moment—we can attempt to maximize the amount of micronutrients we consume on a daily basis. We can only eat so much food in a day, so if we're already dealing with food that's low in micronutrients because of soil quality, we want every bite to count.

"In rough estimates, we consume about two to three pounds of food per day," said Dr. Means. "That means we have two to three pounds per day of opportunity to utilize that molecular material to build the life we want." We've often heard the adage "food is fuel," but thinking of what "fuel" truly means from a scientific perspective is perhaps a more motivating and certainly more research-backed reframe. Every bite is an opportunity for both pleasure (a core component of eating, according to Dr. Means, and one I obviously heartily endorse), but also to consume the micronutrients that create ATP, our body's fuel. "I want to maximize the limited number of calories and quantity of food I have today to serve what my real goals and interests are—long-term contentment and health," explained Dr. Means.

Throughout your day, look for little opportunities to swap in or add more micronutrient-rich foods—typically this involves adding in foods that are rich in vitamins and minerals, or swapping ultra-processed foods for their less processed counterparts. Top your oatmeal with nuts and seeds. When it's within budget, purchase grass-fed or pasture-raised animal protein that was raised on healthy soil. Try to swap ultraprocessed foods for foods that are as close in form to how they were grown as possible, because the steps of processing often result in micronutrient depletion—think of using farro or wild rice as a whole-grain base for meals, or if you're choosing between, say, cracker brands, looking for the nut- and seed-rich one. And, of course, since produce is still one of the most micronutrient-rich foods, use as many plants as possible as the building blocks for your daily diet. Shop at your farmers' market whenever you can, because the food you find there is often grown on richer, better cared for soil, and as such will be more micronutrient rich (you can always ask at the stall about the farm's growing practices!).

Bite for bite, start to consider maximizing micronutrients. Give your car the power it needs to get you exactly where you want to go.

68.

Floss (and tongue scrape!).

You know you should floss. You've heard it a million times—I had, certainly, but it wasn't until a few years ago that I actually made it a regular habit. The key was realizing that flossing wasn't only critical for the health of my teeth (which are important, obviously, but less motivating for me personally than my dentist would prefer), but for the health of my entire body.

"The microbiome in our mouth and inflammation that occurs from things like periodontal disease drives a lot of other inflammatory diseases," explained integrative immunologist Dr. Heather Moday. "There's a link between it and heart disease. There's a link between it and Alzheimer's and brain diseases.[1] We often think we should floss so we don't get cavities, but we don't think of the mouth microbiome and the state of the health of our gums and our teeth as affecting other organs, specifically things like the heart and your brain."

In fact, a well-trained dentist can discern critical information about the health of your entire body simply by looking in your mouth. "Periodontal disease is essentially a cytokine response,"[2] explained Dr. Mark Burhenne, a functional dentist and author of *The 8-Hour Sleep Paradox*. "It's an overreaction of the immune system to a chronic infection in the mouth. But, big picture, it's a severe local inflammatory response, which, then, can seed and aggravate inflammation elsewhere in your body."

This happens through the mechanism of the oral-systemic

connection, Dr. Burhenne explained. "The bugs in the mouth can get into the rest of the body. In the case of Alzheimer's, for example, *P. gingivalis*, the bacteria involved with gum disease, creates a dysbiosis in the mouth that can spread to the bloodstream.[3] Gingipains [a type of enzyme] are produced and cross the blood-brain barrier, causing the brain to lay down amyloid plaque, essentially trying to protect itself from an infection in the mouth!"[4] (In fact, people with poor dental hygiene are 21 percent more likely to develop Alzheimer's disease later in life).[5] Flossing creates mechanical disruption of the plaque that allows the bacteria in the biofilm to reorganize and do their job to protect the teeth and gums, reducing the inflammation and overabundant bacterial colonization.

You want to floss before you brush at least once a day. If you want to take your oral hygiene to the next level, you can add in tongue scraping, a practice that's been used for hundreds of years and studied for its benefits,[6] to get the gunk off your tongue. That gunk is composed of the same bad bacteria that you're getting rid of with the floss. Honestly, all it takes is one time tongue scraping and smelling what comes off to convince you that it's a habit worth keeping—the odors are deeply unpleasant, and somewhat horrifying to imagine in your mouth.

"The tongue is one of the micro niches of the oral microbiome, and if it's feeding a dysbiotic population of bacteria to the rest of the mouth, then all the flossing and brushing of the world is not going to help you," Dr. Burhenne said. "You still want to floss and brush daily, but tongue scraping has its own place in an oral hygiene routine." You can buy affordable tongue scrapers online (mine is stainless steel; I rinse it daily, and run it through the dishwasher once a week or so to deep clean it), and if you're in a pinch, you can also use a spoon. "But you don't want to just use your toothbrush," said Dr. Burhenne. "It's not going to be able to disrupt those bad bacteria."

Do whatever you need to do to make flossing a regular part of your routine, and if you feel inspired, add tongue scraping as well. It's not just for your oral health—it's for your brain and body as well.

69.

Stop snoring.

For my entire life, I thought of snoring as something that's annoying but harmless—I'd giggle in embarrassment if Zack would point out nights that I made a sound he called "a pig hunting for truffles," and count my lucky stars that he was a silent sleeper. And then I started hosting the podcast, and doctor after doctor brought up the dangers of snoring.

"Snoring is not cute. It's not funny, even if your kid does it, or your grandpa does it. It doesn't matter what age and when, if it's infrequent or constant, snoring needs to be addressed," said functional dentist and airway specialist Dr. Mark Burhenne. "It tells you that your airway is collapsing and narrowing, even closing up completely, which wakes you up, because your body won't let you stop breathing or suffocate slowly." Snoring is a symptom of obstructive sleep apnea, and sleep apnea is associated with an increased risk of sudden cardiac death.[1] It's the top-level symptom of your body warning you that it's not getting enough oxygen. It's your body crying for help, and yet many of us laugh and put in some earplugs.

According to Dr. Burhenne, there are other signs you might not be getting the oxygen you need overnight. "There are a lot of unique things that your dentists can see that your physician can't. In fact, I always argue that a dentist can recognize sleep apnea decades before a physician can," he said. "There are some oral signs and symptoms—if you have a scalloped tongue, if you're mouth breathing, if you have a very dry mouth, if you're getting a lot of cavities. You can't take your tongue and push it up and pressurize the top of your palate with your mouth open. But snoring is the big one. My dad snored. My mom snored. I snored. My kids told me I snored. My wife snored. She told me I snored. We did that for fifteen years. It was foolish."

When you fix your snoring, it can fix a whole host of problems you might not even be associating with sleep apnea. "I used to think it was normal to be exhausted all day," Dr. Burhenne said. "I thought it was the process of aging, but when I fixed my sleep apnea, I stopped needing naps. There are a lot of little things that we take for granted that we think are normal, like getting up in the middle of the night and going to the bathroom. That's not always an aging bladder." In fact, research shows sleep apnea increases the secretion of ANP, or atrial natriuretic peptide, at night, which has been found to lead to more frequent urination.[2]

To address potential sleep apnea, you can try at-home steps like getting an air filter or Breathe Right strips to widen your nostrils. Dr. Burhenne is also a fan of mouth taping and using a sleep tracker like an Oura Ring or Apple Watch to help make and track behavioral changes to improve sleep. "Taping, in many incidences, can change the nature of the flow of air past the airway, lessening, even preventing, snoring, or demonstrating that one cannot breathe at all through their nose, even at rest, which would be a clear indicator that professional treatment is needed," Dr. Burhenne said. "And sleep trackers are the best way to figure out the sleep puzzle at home if a sleep study is not affordable or available."

But if the snoring doesn't stop, Dr. Burhenne recommends a polysomnogram (PSG), or attended sleep study. "You want a qualified analysis of your sleep," Dr. Burhenne said. "You want to know how many times you wake up, how many interruptions. To what degree do you have sleep apnea? And why? Do you have central apneas? You want to figure all that out."

First, find out if you snore—if you're not sure, there are apps that can listen for snoring, or you can ask people who have been within listening distance of you as you've slept. Or you can look out for symptoms like a dry mouth in the morning, middle-of-the-night urination, or feeling tired even if you've gotten a full night's sleep. Being unable to successfully mouth tape is also an indicator that your airway is restricted. Next, take steps to address the snoring, whether it's an air filter, dealing with allergies that might clog your nose, seeking out ENTs, orthodontists, dentists, or other airway specialists, or undergoing a sleep study to begin to address the issue.

You wouldn't deny your body food. You wouldn't deny your body water. Stop denying it the air and rest it needs to survive and thrive.

70.

Upgrade the foods
you're already eating.

There are three healthy cooking hacks that I come back to time and again because they don't require adding in any new foods—they simply maximize the potential of what I'm already eating.

The first? Using high-quality olive oil for my cooking and baking. There's a lot of controversy in the "what oil is healthiest?" world, with different types cycling in and out of health-superstar status, in no small part because the media simply needs something new to write about. In my work, I like to look for the common denominators, the health tips that the most experts and doctors seem to agree on and that the most research backs (while recognizing that the nature of science means that research is ever-evolving). When it comes to oils, that point of agreement is olive oil. One of the keys, explained Dr. William Li, an internationally renowned Harvard-trained medical doctor and the author of *Eat to Beat Disease*, is that in general, plants that have to fight to survive produce a lot of bioactives—they are, essentially, the "weapons" the plants use in their quest for their own survival, and some of those weapons can be transferred into *our* arsenal when we eat those plants. "Olive trees grow in really harsh, rocky, dusty climates," said Dr. Li. "That struggle to even grow there creates a lot of bioactives."

One of the bioactives that has a lot of research behind it is a polyphenol called hydroxytyrosol. "When we used hydroxytyrosol in the lab, we found it actually killed cancer cells and cut off the blood supply feeding cancers as well," said Dr. Li. "It also helped protect stem cells." There's ample research that associates olive oil with lower risk of heart disease,[1] and studies have pointed to its beneficial effect on our gut microbiome.[2] And while I don't think historical use always makes something healthy or worth doing (our ancestors' choices were often the result of their circumstances and are not always applicable to our modern world), I do think that the use of olive oil over thousands of years by some of the longest-lived people in the world is a vote in its favor.

When you're shopping for olive oil, always look for "extra-virgin" on the label; anything else indicates a lower-quality product that will both taste worse and have fewer benefits. While it's not a requirement, looking for a third-party certification seal can also be a helpful indicator of quality: the European Union's protected designation of origin (PDO) seal or the "Certified Extra Virgin" seal from the California Olive Oil Council for California-made oils are both good ones to seek out. Interestingly, one of the best ways to tell if you're getting good-quality olive oil is simply by tasting it: it should taste grassy, fresh, and a little peppery, and the more antioxidant-rich it is, the more it'll create the sensation that you have to cough at the back of your throat.

If you want to take it to the next level and absolutely maximize the amount of polyphenols you get from your olive oil—which also contains oleocanthal, luteolin, and apigenin, all of which have researched anticancer and antidisease effects[3]—but you get overwhelmed by all the options at the store, Dr. Li shared a fun trick: "Look for monovarietal olive oils, or oils made with only one type of olive," he said. "There are three varieties of olives that generate oil with the highest levels of polyphenols: Greek olive oil made with Koroneiki olives; Spanish olive oil made with Picual olives; and Italian olive oil made with Moraiolo olives." This will be indicated on the bottle; it'll always say if it's monovarietal, and typically will indicate the country of origin if not the exact olive type.

While there's been some worry about cooking with olive oil, the studies don't support a need for concern: it has a smoke point

between 374° and 405°F, which is adequate for the vast majority
of home cooking. While, like many foods, it might lose some of
its benefits when exposed to heat, numerous studies have shown
that it doesn't form harmful compounds. In fact, because of all of
its antioxidants and its high levels of oleic acid, olive oil actually
keeps its nutritional value better than most other oils when used
for cooking with heat.[4]

The second trick? Resting your garlic. Chopping garlic acti-
vates an enzyme called alliinase, which converts the alliin natu-
rally present in fresh garlic to a compound called allicin.[5] Allicin
is absolutely rife with benefits—studies have found it to be antivi-
ral, antifungal, antiparasitic, and antibacterial[6] (it's been shown
to even kill antibiotic-resistant strains of bacteria![7]). It's also been
found to *help* the beneficial bacteria in our gut,[8] while targeting
the problematic ones—a win.

Once present, allicin is incredibly delicate, and can be destroyed
by exposure to heat and oxygen (which means, unfortunately, that
the prechopped garlic available at the grocery store has likely lost
most of its allicin content). My favorite tactic is to chop the gar-
lic I need at the beginning of making a recipe, then let it sit while
I'm prepping everything else. Then I modify the recipe to add the
garlic just at the end, cooking it for 1 to 2 minutes, max, to dull
its sharp flavor (which can otherwise overwhelm the balance of a
dish) without destroying the heat-sensitive allicin. (If I'm ever feel-
ing sick, I also make my go-to garlic toast: chopped, rested garlic
on toast with olive oil, any dried herbs I have on hand, and a little
bit of sea salt.)

Lastly, I let my cruciferous vegetables sit for 40 minutes to acti-
vate their epinutrients, the nutrients that impact whether certain
genes in the body get turned "on" or "off." Research shows that
consuming sulforaphane, which is found in broccoli and cruci-
ferous vegetables, can help reduce the epigenetic damage caused
by smoking,[9] an effect that was also shown in terms of mitigating
air pollution. "Scientists measured how much DNA damage these
people received, and after supplementation with epinutrients, part

of this damage was undone," said Stanford epigeneticist Dr. Lucia Aronica.[10]

Sulforaphane is produced as a reaction to chewing or chopping the vegetables,[11] which brings us back to our amazingly simple hack: after chopping your cruciferous veggies, let them sit. "Pre-chopping the cruciferous vegetable lets more sulforaphane develop, which is advantageous, because more is better in the first place, and also because sulforaphane is less heat-sensitive than myrosinase, so you can cook the vegetable more with less epinutrient die-off," said Dr. Aronica.

When you have time, chop cruciferous vegetables—including broccoli, watercress, cauliflower, kohlrabi, arugula, Brussels sprouts, cabbage, kale, mustard greens, radishes, rutabagas, turnips—and let them sit for 40 minutes before you cook. Sulforaphane is reduced when exposed to heat, so I also try to diversify my veggie prep. If I've been eating a lot of kale chips, I'll incorporate a lightly sautéed massaged kale salad; watercress is delicious raw or lightly sautéed.

Finally, if you want to increase the nutrient value of your cruciferous veggies even more, pair them with mustard. "Mustard seeds contain the myrosinase enzyme," said Dr. Aronica, "which helps to produce more sulforaphane."[12] I like to make a mustard vinaigrette for my arugula salads, or to use whole mustard seeds to add crunch, zest, and extra health benefits to broccoli, cauliflower, and Brussels sprout dishes.

Again, I don't use all three tricks (or even one of them) every time I eat; rather, they sit in the back of my mind so that I can easily incorporate one when I think of it or have the time, an easy way to get more goodness out of what I'm already consuming.

71.

Challenge limiting aging beliefs.

When you become aware of negative aging beliefs, a glass shatters, and suddenly, you'll notice them *everywhere*—on greeting cards, in conversations with your friends, in jokes on TV. It's pervasive, and it starts *young*—I regularly get messages from women in their thirties and even mid- to late twenties who are worried they're getting "old."

The problem with these limiting aging beliefs is that they're not true, they're largely seeded by people with a vested interest in taking your money and/or power, and they literally steal years from your life—7.5 years, to be exact,[1] according to a study by Yale professor Dr. Becca Levy, a leading researcher in the psychology of aging and author of *Breaking the Age Code*.

In this groundbreaking study, her team found that the *single most important factor* (above gender, income, social background, loneliness, and functional health) in determining longevity was how people felt about and approached aging. So that silly postcard about being "over the hill"? That friend joking about your group being too old for a night out or a hike? They're seeding and normalizing beliefs that are costing you years of your life.

The first step in breaking free from these negative aging beliefs is to start to become aware of the negative aging messages you're internalizing from outside sources—and the ones you're telling yourself. "There's a tendency to automatically blame aging for our health problems as we get older," said Dr. Levy. "Let's say you have an ache in your back, and your first thought is, 'I must be getting old.' But really, it could be due to something else entirely—maybe you were shoveling the day before or doing a new exercise."

Dr. Levy encourages people to think about alternative explanations for symptoms they're experiencing—can you not hear because your hearing is declining, or is it just that the restaurant is loud? Does your knee hurt because your joints are degrading, or because you walked a lot yesterday? "Try to think about whether there are different ways to explain health challenges that aren't attributable to aging," she said.

At the same time, call out the negative aging messages that show up from others on a day-to-day basis. When my friends say, "We're too old to go out dancing," I reply, "Says who? I love dancing." While they might seem innocuous, these tiny comments add up, and they're shaping both our beliefs and our longevity.

Another one of Dr. Levy's favorite ways to combat negative aging beliefs is to develop a portfolio of positive aging role models. "Everybody has these positive images of aging that they've encountered, but they're not always at the forefront in our mind when we think about aging," she shared. "If I ask people, 'What are five words or phrases that come to mind when you think of an old person?,' which is a question I've used in a number of studies, we find that in the United States, most times, the first images people mention are often negative. But by the time they get to their fourth or fifth example, they often are positive."

The trick, then, lies in how we strengthen those positive images so they're more in the forefront of our minds when we think about aging. "Come up with four or five examples of positive images or portrayals of older people," Dr. Levy said. "They could be from your own family, a favorite book that you've read, or a TV show. With each example, then think about two qualities of that person that you admire and that you would like to strengthen in yourself."

I've intentionally followed positive aging role models on social media—I look for women who are living lives rich in travel and relationships, who are relishing new beginnings and opportunities at all phases of their lives. I've also sought out positive aging role models in the professional world, from a woman who made a career pivot in her forties and went on to become a *New York Times* bestselling author, to my aunt, who, in her fifties, became the CEO of a now thriving company working to fight climate change. Surrounding myself with these examples has subconsciously shifted my beliefs about what's possible as I grow older. Of course, a successful life means something different to all of us, so be on the lookout for people you find personally inspiring. Follow them on social media, keep a list on your phone, make collages for your desk, or make a scrapbook that you can revisit as needed.

By taking a stance against aging, our society has imbued with negativity the single inevitable element of human existence. While it's perhaps not surprising—it can feel quite insidious if you consider that if every person must age and we create a world that hates aging, we create an inexhaustible well of consumers—it's not serving us.

Take your power back. The one thing that no one can argue about aging is that it *is*, and we can't change that—but we *can* change our beliefs about what it means, and in doing so add years to our lives.

72.

Reassess your relationship with alcohol.

This one took me a long time to hear, and I think it's a message that comes to you when you're ready for it. For years, I've asked doctors and researchers: What's the best type of alcohol to drink if you're concerned about your health? What's the best way to drink it? And each time, whether we were talking about longevity, cancer, hormones, the gut, the brain, or even the skin, the answer came back crystal clear: for your health, the *best* amount of alcohol to drink is none.

Yet I kept drinking. I ate well, I worked out, I meditated. How much harm could a few glasses of champagne cause? Never content with simply asking an open-ended question, I decided to do everything in my power to find out. I put together a podcast series about the health impacts of alcohol, and interviewed top doctors and experts. The results were, well, sobering.

Research shows that alcohol consumption is one of the biggest risk factors for cancer, along with smoking.[1] It weakens our defenses against viruses[2] and causes irreparable mutations in our stem cells.[3] It causes acid reflux[4] and dehydration,[5] and blocks our ability to get REM and deep sleep.[6] It raises the level of fat in the blood,[7] which can increase risk of heart disease, and can impair GABA balance in the brain,[8] increasing mental health concerns like anxiety and depression. It's been linked, even in the smallest amounts, to an increased risk of breast cancer.[9]

Having this information made me look at alcohol differently. Were the results I was experiencing actually worth the harm I was causing to my body? Was it actually enhancing my life, on net? I stopped drinking almost entirely then, and found out that, in fact, it wasn't. Because we're all *already* the person we think alcohol is making us. All alcohol does is lower our inhibitions so we let that person come out. If you dance for hours on end when you're drinking, *you are already* that dancer. If you're witty and charming, *you are already* that delightful conversationalist. If you think you're gorgeous when you're drunk, *you are already* that stunning person. The alcohol just let you silence your inner critic so those parts of yourself could come out without fear of rejection.

Moreover, not drinking hasn't been nearly as awkward or embarrassing as I thought it would be. If someone judges you for not drinking—well, isn't that embarrassing for *them*? Why do they care so much? I also find that there's an initial hump, right at the beginning of a night out or social gathering, where everyone is ordering drinks and loosening up and I have to use my own mental resources to relax and get into that conversational flow. But once that happens, I'm *set*. I'm off to the races, ready to be a sparkling conversationalist for the rest of the evening, while *everyone else* is getting more cognitively impaired. I actually find people enjoy spending time out with me *more* now, because I'm able to bring more to the table. Not drinking has also been an encouragement to be more creative with the time I spend with friends, resulting in game nights filled with belly-aching laughter, cookbook potluck parties, and outdoor adventures. I've also found new ways to relax after work that leave me feeling truly restored, relaxed, and ready to take on the next day (see box, page 268).

I'm not going to be the one to tell you to give up alcohol entirely (unless, of course, you're dealing with addiction, in which case, please work with a professional healthcare provider). In fact, most of the doctors I interviewed about the health impacts of alcohol for my podcast series said they still drank on occasion, usually when some type of ritual was involved, and even I am not opposed to having a drink here and there, when and if I feel the urge—I've personally found dogmatic rules can lead to disordered thoughts when it comes to my health.

But I do think it's worth considering your own equation—what are the negatives? And do the positives make up for it? When I stopped drinking, I was myopically focused on everything I was giving up, in the name of gaining an abstract notion of health. But what I've found is the opposite—I've gained deeper friendships, more energy, less anxiety, and literally days of my life that I would've spent hungover (when I first stopped drinking, doing the calculation that I was losing almost a month of my year to hangovers was a starkly motivating exercise).

Maybe you experiment with having a mocktail or another fun drink next time you're out, and let yourself begin to gather those proof points that you're already the sparkly person you think alcohol is making you, that you *can* have fun without it. Maybe you try a few days of skipping that after-work drink. Whatever you do, there's enough research at this point to support approaching alcohol with significantly more intentionality, and figuring out what place it truly deserves to occupy in your life.

WANT TO DIVE DEEPER?

Listen to these episodes of The Liz Moody Podcast:

- "Ask the Doctor: Immune Health Edition—Lower Inflammation, Reduce Allergies & Spend Less Time Being Sick with Heather Moday, MD," episode 101

- "Ask the Doctor: Dental Health Edition—Fluoride, Whitening & How Your Oral Health Impacts Your Gut, Heart, and More with Mark Burhenne, DDS," episode 75

- "What to Eat for Longevity, Inflammation, Cancer Prevention, Alzheimer's, Diabetes, & More with Dr. William Li," episode 124

- "Ask the Doctor: Epigenetics Edition—How to Hack Your Genes to Increase Lifespan, Reverse Cellular Damage, & Fight Disease with Dr. Lucia Aronica," episode 135

- "Busting Myths About Aging: Live Longer and Feel Better with Dr. Becca Levy," episode 107

- "The Health Effects of Alcohol: Gut Health & Cancer with Dr. Robynne Chutkan & Dr. William Li," episode 153

- "The Health Effects of Alcohol: Hormones & Brain Health with Dr. Aviva Romm & Louisa Nicola," episode 154

- "How to Drink Less Without Feeling Boring, Judged, or Stressed with Amanda E. White, LPC," episode 155

Explore these resources from our expert guests:

- *The Immunotype Breakthrough: Your Personalized Plan to Balance Your Immune System, Optimize Health, and Build Lifelong Resistance* by Dr. Heather Moday, @theimmunitymd on Instagram

- *The 8-Hour Sleep Paradox: How We Are Sleeping Our Way to Fatigue, Disease & Unhappiness* by Dr. Mark Burhenne, www .askthedentist.com

- *Eat to Beat Disease: The New Science of How Your Body Can Heal Itself* by Dr. William Li, www.drwilliamli.com

- Dr. Lucia Aronica, www.draronica.com

- *Breaking the Age Code: How Your Beliefs About Aging Determine How Long & Well You Live* by Dr. Becca Levy, www.becca-levy.com

- *Hormone Intelligence: The Complete Guide to Calming Hormone Chaos and Restoring Your Body's Natural Blueprint for Well-Being* by Dr. Aviva Romm, www.avivaromm.com

HOW TO
FEEL CALMER

73.

Set a news boundary.

One practice that almost every doctor and expert I've interviewed has in common? A solid boundary around the news. While these folks are all active and engaged citizens, they also recognize that much of the news we consume is designed as entertainment, not need-to-know information—which means it's specifically created to elicit the types of emotional reactions that get more clicks or watch-time.

Start by having an honest conversation with yourself about whether you're learning information that you *need* to know or simply using media apps to kill time (time that you could be filling with your "Life Is Never Boring" activities, per page 159, or even using to just do nothing, per page 93), or consuming news to feel a sense of control over things that are out of your control (when you could be applying an activist mindset and actually creating change in the world that in turn cultivates calm in your body, per page 254).

Then see what boundaries you can set that could turn you into a more intentional news consumer. I know, for instance, that when I watch television news, I get anxious and overstimulated, and much prefer to get my news via podcast or long-form media. Is there a time of day that the news feels more helpful and less harmful in your life? Personally, if I start the day with the news, I can end up in a spiral of despair. I'm not productive, I don't achieve what I want to achieve, and guess what? The world isn't made any better by my actions.

One of the doctors I interviewed receives all her news from her partner, who acts as a filter, while another eschews articles and prefers to only consume nonfiction books for a more zoomed-out, thought-through view; still another sets aside fifteen minutes every morning (he even uses a timer!) to cycle through his favorite apps while he drinks his coffee.

The only *wrong* way to consume news is without intention, and unfortunately, that's what many of us end up doing. Is it entertaining you if it's making you feel depressed and anxious? Is it "good to be informed" when that information regularly leaves you in a state of flight or freeze so you can't actually take the actions in your life that would make the information beneficial?

I'm not suggesting that you live with your head in the sand and ignore the real and scary things happening in the world. I'm suggesting that your attention is one of your most precious resources, and many of us have let ours be hijacked, thinking we're doing something good for ourselves or the world, when really the result is counterproductive both inwardly and outwardly.

Evaluate your relationship with the news. What are your goals around news consumption? How can you alter your habits to help you meet those goals? Set boundaries to expose yourself to information in a way that helps you be both the person and the citizen you want to be.

74.

Do a life-admin day.

Sometimes stress or anxiety comes from a real emotional place. Sometimes it comes from false moods (see page 258). And sometimes it comes from simply having too many small, nagging things on your to-do list.

That's where a life-admin day comes in. On a life-admin day, you make a list of all those little items that have been occupying the corners of your brain: returning packages, replying to emails or texts, running errands, breaking down boxes, making doctor's appointments, folding that pile of laundry that's been sitting there for weeks . . . You can also use a life-admin day to kick off projects you've been procrastinating on, since the weight of knowing you need to start something can be heavy. Is there an upcoming presentation or report or homework assignment that you've been putting off? A vacation you need to make reservations for? I actually began the project of writing this book on a life-admin day.

Start your life-admin day by doing a brain dump of everything that's occupying the nooks and crannies of your mind, and consider each individual item. If there's a task that can be completed immediately, get it done (I kick off my life-admin day with an easy win, because objects in motion stay in motion, per page 99). If it's something that's going to take a little longer, just get it started. Getting over that initial hurdle is often far more impactful than we think.

I like to do a life-admin day every two weeks or so, and I try to make it feel as fun as possible: I temptation bundle (see page 28) by listening to my favorite podcasts and treating myself to a favorite tea or mocktail. At the end of the day, I feel as refreshed as if I had done a meditation session or massage—if not more. Sometimes, we need to relieve stress in our minds. Thinking about the same thing on your to-do list over and over and over again can create its own kind of decision fatigue (see page 61). Eliminating those tangible sources of stress in our lives can give us space to do so much more.

If you can't do a life-admin day, can you schedule in a life-admin afternoon? A life-admin hour? Find an amount of time and cadence that works for you, and stick to it. Whatever your unique tasks are, use dedicated life-admin time to get them done and free up the space they're occupying in your mind.

75.

Meditate—but for less time than you think.

It probably doesn't surprise you that the experts I've spoken with over the years consistently cite meditation as one of their top recommended tools. What *might* surprise you is the amount of time they say you need to meditate in order to reap the benefits.

"At NYU, the shortest experiment we've run was with a five-minute visual meditation, and it was shown to significantly decrease immediate anxiety levels," said Dr. Wendy Suzuki, a professor of neuroscience and psychology at NYU and the author of *Good Anxiety*. Her lab is continuing to explore the effects of even shorter amounts of meditation to determine the absolute minimum dose that still effectively reduces stress and offers health benefits.

Dr. Amishi Jha, a psychology professor at the University of Miami who studies focus and attention, had a similar experience. "In our work with pre-deployment military service members, we were like, 'They're busy people, let's just ask them to do thirty minutes a day,'" she said. "Very few people did thirty minutes a day. So I went back and said, 'Let's be honest. What did you actually do?'

"That number looked like about twelve minutes a day," she said. "In subsequent studies, we didn't even ask them to do thirty minutes, and we noticed many more people were willing to comply." They asked participants to meditate every day, and again experienced low compliance, so they experimented with the fewest possible days required to see results. Now Dr. Jha's lab prescribes twelve to fifteen minutes a day, three to five times a week to see the benefits in terms of focus and attention.

Parsley Health founder Dr. Robin Berzin tells her patients to incorporate meditation throughout their day, in any way that feels good to them, in increments that are manageable—whether that's two, five, or ten minutes at a time. "Run away from anyone who tells you that their way to meditate is the only way. There are a million ways to meditate and almost all of them are good. You can meditate while you're taking a walk. You can meditate on your commute," she said. "You don't need a mantra. You don't need a fancy cushion. You can just inhale for four, exhale for six. When you breathe longer on the exhale, you stimulate the vagus nerve and induce a parasympathetic state."[1]

While Dr. Berzin's practice and Dr. Jha's and Dr. Suzuki's research were focused on different desired outcomes, they all highlight a need to set the bar significantly lower. I encounter so many people who express a desire to meditate, but have trouble deciding what to do and sticking to a routine. In my mind, Dr. Suzuki's and Dr. Jha's research and Dr. Berzin's words serve as a permission slip to commit to a much more reasonable practice.

Lowering the bar in terms of how you *feel* is also key to creating and maintaining a consistent practice. The experience of meditation isn't always ease and bliss. In fact, I've found the first few minutes of meditation often make me *more* anxious; it's like that moment when you're cleaning and everything gets *more* chaotic before ending up in its proper place. Feeling anxious or antsy or stressed during a session doesn't mean you're doing it wrong; in fact, it's a sign that you *need* this practice.

You also don't need to be free from distracted thoughts for meditation to be effective. A teacher of mine once described the practice as similar to weight lifting: every time your mind wanders away and you bring it back, that's a rep. The *practice* isn't sitting there with a completely clear mind, but rather bringing *back* your wandering mind, over and over again. It's not a personal flaw or failing—you're experiencing the essence of what meditation *is*.

Don't beat yourself up for any emotions that surface. Don't berate yourself for thinking about your breakfast, or a work meeting, or that argument you had with your partner. Just gently bring your mind back to whatever you're focusing on. That is the practice. Look at you! You're meditating!

Start with five minutes a day. Don't make it fancy—you can go on Spotify, YouTube, or Insight Timer and find thousands of free options for guided meditations, or you can just set a timer and say a mantra or follow your breath for five minutes. If five minutes feels good, after a month or two, make it ten minutes. Build up to Dr. Jha's twelve minute sessions and see if you start noticing differences in your ability to direct your attention where you want it to be.

But just five minutes counts, I promise. And by trying to do more, we often end up not doing anything at all, and experiencing none of the myriad benefits.

76.

Use action as the antidote to anxiety.

If there's one sentence that has fundamentally changed my approach to my anxiety, it's this: action is the antidote to anxiety. Read that again: action is the antidote to anxiety. It's come up a few times in my conversations—first with *Radically Content* author Jamie Varon, who spoke to the shame components of inaction: "Fear multiplies when we're not doing the thing that we want to be doing. It becomes this monster. Action cures fear." Every bit of action takes away some of the unknown, and builds confidence in your ability to handle whatever comes your way.

In fact, action is what anxiety is *designed* to produce. "Anxiety has evolved to activate us," explained neuroscientist Dr. Wendy Suzuki. "It looks a little bit different in the modern world—we're not running away or fighting a lion. But our anxiety evolved to have an actionable outcome. That's the thing that helps resolve the anxiety."

Today, think of one thing you're anxious or stressed about, and then think of one action—however small—you could take related to that thing. If you're anxious about an upcoming project, spend five minutes working on it. If you're anxious about the state of a relationship, send that person a text. If you're anxious about a health outcome, schedule a doctor's appointment. If you're anxious about the state of the world, make a donation to a cause you believe in or set up a time to volunteer in your local community. I've been applying this philosophy for over a year now, and I've found there's always *an* action I can take related to the thing causing me anxiety, and I always, *always* feel better once I take it. What's one action you can take today?

77.

Stop letting fear control your relationship with money.

One of the simplest ways to transform your life is to master the concept of knowing what's in your control and what's out of it. It's a practice I return to again and again, as I find myself fretting about a political headline or a fight I've had with my husband (and applying an activist mindset to what's in our control is one of the best ways to assuage our anxiety; see page 254).

In various studies, money comes out as a top, if not *the* top, source of stress[1] in our lives, again and again—yet few of us actually take the time to truly consider what parts of our financial situation are within our control. "People are always asking me, 'What's going to happen next in the market? What's going on with inflation? What about a recession?'" said financial expert Ramit Sethi when I interviewed him. "The truth is, nobody knows what's going to happen, so you should stop putting your faith in a person. Whether they're on CNBC or it's me—stop. Many people are looking for some parental figure to reassure them, 'It's going to be okay.' It's never coming. Take control of your money. You need to understand how personal finance works."

I spent years laughing about what I called my avoidant attachment style with money, co-opted from the psychological relationship concept of attachment theory. Wasn't it funny that I didn't know about investing? Wasn't it just so "me" to tune out when it came to tax talk?

My conversation with Sethi made me realize that it wasn't cute, it wasn't charming, and it wasn't contributing to my overall sense of happiness or well-being. "There are so many people who are scared of investing," Sethi said. "But these are the same people who have never read a single book about personal finance."

I realized that in all the time I spent worrying about the overall economy—something I have very little control over—I devoted very little learning to my *own* finances, something very much within my control.

I've learned that today, I can take one step toward financial wellness in an area that is within my control. I can read a personal finance book (Sethi's is amazing). I can set up a target date index fund and put some money into it. (Another secret I've learned from personal finance experts: Good investing is not about picking individual stocks, but rather just sticking your money in distributed funds and not touching it for years. It's boring, but that's it—that's the whole thing.) I can follow a variety of personal finance experts on social media so I can learn from them without taking on their opinions as indisputable facts.

The next time your focus slips into money anxiety that's out of your control, bring your mind back to the money choices you *do* have the ability to make—there are more of them than you think. Your wallet and mental health will thank you.

78.

Limit the physical causes of anxiety.

Have you ever felt *deeply, truly* annoyed with a person—and then you ate a snack, and suddenly, the powerful emotions barely resonated anymore? That, explained Yale- and Columbia-trained psychiatrist Dr. Ellen Vora, is a false mood.

According to Dr. Vora, many of our moods, from anxiety to anger, can be attributed not just to what's going on in our mind, but to what's going on in our body. "Your blood sugar is crashing, or you're hungover and you're in a GABA withdrawal state, or you're inflamed, or sleep-deprived. These physical states can make you feel sad or anxious," she said. "Sometimes, your moods aren't about the world being terrible or hating your partner. Sometimes, your physiology is out of balance, your body is in a stress response, and it's creating a feeling like anxiety."

There are a few things Dr. Vora recommends to limit the harmful effects of false moods, and the first is just paying attention. "Keep a list on the refrigerator of the false moods you find yourself dipping into so you can identify them in the moment of anxiety," Dr. Vora said. "It's similar to having a newborn baby, where you have to be like: 'Why are they fussy? Is it a wet diaper? Are they hungry? Are they tired? Do they need to be burped?' You have to learn the system: 'Why is the baby fussy?' Or in the case of false anxiety: 'Why is the grown-up fussy?'"

Blood sugar is one of the key false anxieties that Dr. Vora recommends paying attention to. "In my experience, anxiety is a blood sugar issue until proven otherwise—meaning anxiety often tracks with blood sugar crashes. That's actually good news, because it's a form of anxiety that is eminently fixable," she said. "Given that many of our diets are built on a foundation of refined carbohydrates, coffee drinks that are secretly milkshakes, and rosé all day, we often run around on a blood sugar roller coaster, spiking and then crashing."

That blood sugar crash creates a stress response in the body, as our stress hormones—cortisol and adrenaline—cue the liver to break down its glycogen stores to bring our blood sugar back to baseline. "That's the system of checks and balances to prevent our organs from failing due to low blood sugar," Dr. Vora explained. "It saves the day, but it leaves us rattled, because we just had a five-alarm fire in the body. A blood sugar crash produces a stress response, and a stress response can feel synonymous with anxiety and panic for some people."

To start to take control of your blood sugar, you can learn how to prepare metabolically optimized meals (see page 49) and make small tweaks like going for walks or doing squats after meals (see page 59). Dr. Vora is also a fan of having a spoonful of nut butter to blunt a blood sugar crash in a pinch. You can also eat some before bed to keep your blood sugar steady overnight, which can be helpful if you find yourself waking up in the middle of the night (that 3 a.m. wake-up with racing thoughts can point to many things, including sleep apnea, per page 231, but can also be caused by low blood sugar).

Hormonal cycles can be another cause of false moods. I track my menstrual cycle for a number of reasons, but being able to open the app that one time of the month when I suddenly want to break up with Zack, quit my job, move towns, and/or lie under a blanket on the couch all day, and find that my period is coming in a few days is incredibly helpful. Now if I feel like everything is horrible or I want to make a huge change during that window, I can remind myself that in a few days, I'll likely feel much better—and if I don't,

I'll have more clarity and information and be better positioned to make the real changes my life requires.

Again—none of this is to say feelings aren't valid. They 100 percent are—and knowing where they're coming from, whether the root is physical or emotional, is the first step toward addressing those feelings. But according to Dr. Vora, "Sometimes our anxious thoughts are simply our minds trying to make sense of what is first and foremost a physical sensation. We can address false anxiety at the level of the body, and eliminate a lot of unnecessary suffering." Think about it this way: if you can address 50 percent of your anxiety by keeping your blood sugar balanced, it not only massively enhances your life, it frees up so much mental space and energy to begin to tackle the other 50 percent.

Get familiar with your false anxiety triggers. When you feel anxious, take a moment to explore what else might be going on. Are you hungry? What's your hormonal state? Have you been sleeping well? Do you have too much on your plate and need a life-admin day (see page 249)? Keep a list on your fridge like Dr. Vora suggests, or on your phone, and begin to address what might lie beneath your feelings.

79.

Try a breathwork practice.

My father is a psychologist, and he's been touting the benefits of box breathing for my entire life. He often works with clients who have limited resources to support their mental health, and starting a breathwork practice–which is free, and can be done in almost all environments–is one of his top recommendations for them.

Our autonomic functions manage the automatic parts of our bodies that we need to survive–everything going on that you aren't consciously aware of, like your heartbeat, your digestion, and your ability to sweat. Breathing is unique because it's the only part of the autonomic system that you can control–meaning that while the vast majority of the time, you're breathing without thinking, you *can* also modify your breath, causing cascading effects on the rest of your body.

Many of those benefits are created via the suppression of the sympathetic nervous system and the activation of the parasympathetic nervous system, which is also referred to as the "rest and digest" branch of your nervous system. "Your fight-or-flight system ramps up cortisol," explained NYU neuroscience professor Dr. Wendy Suzuki. "When the danger disappears, your parasympathetic system kicks in to help you relax." This is typically achieved by slowing down your breath and elongating your exhales. "Slow conscious breathing, which is part of normal parasympathetic activation, can jump-start the entire system," Dr. Suzuki explained. "It decreases heart rate. It brings blood back into your digestive and reproductive systems. And it begins to reduce your anxiety on a neurological level."

A recent Stanford study pitted mindfulness meditation against cyclic sighing, box breathing, and cyclic hyperventilation and found that while all groups experienced positive effects, including reduced stress and improved mood, all three of the breathwork groups experienced greater improvements, with cyclic sighing having the greatest positive effects.[1]

We're at the tip of the iceberg when it comes to understanding the many ways we can impact our body via our breath, but the research is clear: the effects are powerful. If you'd like to experiment with a breathwork practice, my two favorites are cyclic sighing and box breathing.

To practice a cyclic or physiological sigh, take two sniffs through your nose, hold briefly, and follow with one long exhale through your mouth. Repeat 2 or 3 times. This is the breathwork practice that was found to be the most effective in the Stanford study.[2] It slows your heart rate, and I've found fairly instantly reduces feelings of stress and anxiety.

Box breathing has also been shown to be a powerful activator of the parasympathetic nervous system. To do it, just breathe in through your nose for a count of 4, hold it for a count of 4, breathe out for a count of 4, and hold for another count of 4 (effectively creating 4 counts of 4, or a "box").

I also love the app Breathwrk, which has breathwork practices for a variety of goals (calm, focus, energy) that you can do in as little as a minute.

There are two ways to incorporate this tip: either begin a daily practice to reduce overall stress, or use breathwork as a tool in moments that you need it. I find a combination of both works well— I do an exercise on Breathwrk daily, and then will come back to cyclic sighing or box breathing in times that I feel particularly stressed or anxious. I also love to use it when my brain is racing at night to help clear some of that frenetic energy and slip into a state where I can relax into sleep, which is a technique endorsed by sleep scientist Vanessa Hill. It feels wildly powerful to be able to change my state in a noticeable physiological and psychological way in less time than it takes to make a cup of tea or send an email.

Whatever you choose, the first step is simply the awareness that our breath is free, quick, easy to access, and discreet (no one needs to know if you're utilizing it)—and it's one of the most powerful tools at our disposal for changing both our psychological and physiological state.

WANT TO DIVE DEEPER?

Listen to these episodes of **The Liz Moody Podcast:**
- "How to Use Neuroscience to Eliminate Anxiety, Become More Optimistic, and Overcome Childhood Trauma with Dr. Wendy Suzuki," episode 83
- "Ask the Doctor: Anxiety Edition—Everything You Need to Know About Treating Anxiety Naturally with Ellen Vora, MD," episode 36
- Ask the Doctor: Burn Out Edition—How to Get Back Your Energy & Eliminate Overwhelm with Dr. Robin Berzin," episode 96

Explore these resources from our expert guests:
- *Good Anxiety: Harnessing the Power of the Most Misunderstood Emotion* by Dr. Wendy Suzuki, www.wendysuzuki.com
- *The Anatomy of Anxiety: Understanding and Overcoming the Body's Fear Response* by Dr. Ellen Vora, @ellenvoramd on Instagram
- *State Change: End Anxiety, Beat Burnout, and Ignite a New Baseline of Energy and Flow* by Dr. Robin Berzin, www.parsley health.com

HOW TO
RESTORE AND RESET

80

Have a post-work ritual.

I struggle with my work life bleeding into my evening time, a struggle that's becoming increasingly typical as hybrid work and working from home become more common. There are the obvious forms of work creeping into your personal time, like sitting down to answer emails after dinner, but there are also more subtle ways that it slips in, whether it's a problem we can't stop thinking about or a stressed mood that lingers.

If creating a boundary between work and home is an issue for you, you might benefit from creating a post-work ritual. Our brains aren't built to effortlessly switch from work mode to social mode, and creating a ritual that marks the end of one and the beginning of another can help it make that transition. While changing your external world can seem trivial, it's actually one of the most powerful ways to change the state of our brains. I'm guilty of ignoring this: when I'm in a bad mood, it can feel like cheating to go on a walk or eat something that gives me energy or take a shower. I need to address the root of my bad mood, not mask it! But in fact, it's all a tangled web: our external factors trigger our moods, which can have cascading effects on our hormones and neurology, which can then trigger new moods and so on. Changing your external state isn't a Band-Aid, but a powerful way to disrupt the cycle before it even begins.

Numerous studies point to the benefits of having a defined workspace, which is increasingly hard as more of us work from home. At a bare minimum, I designate a place for my computer to sit; when my work is done for the day, I close my laptop and put it on a shelf instead of leaving it out on the kitchen table where it can catch my eye and attention for the rest of the evening. I'm also a huge fan of showering or taking a walk once the laptop is closed, again, looking to alter my psychology by altering my physiology.

I've included a few more ideas below—use them as inspiration, or pick something else that resonates with you. Whatever you choose, use it to draw a clear mental boundary between work and home, so you can benefit from the restorative time you deserve.

POST-WORK RITUAL IDEAS

- Change from work clothes into comfy clothes.

- Have a standing phone or in-person date with a friend.

- Close your computer and put it in a different room.

- Put on a relaxing playlist and light a candle.

- Put on an energizing playlist and dance around.

- Make a pot of tea.

- Make a cocktail or mocktail.

- Do a ten-minute journaling session.

- Meditate.

- Have an intentional play session with your child or pet.

- Get in a quick workout.

- Make a snack.

81.

Give your brain a bath.

While the type of yoga that involves sweaty classes filled with people contorting their bodies into pose after pose looms large in Western culture, there are actually many types of yoga—and yoga nidra is one that involves as *little* movement as possible.

Neuroscientist Dr. Tara Swart Bieber explained that yoga nidra is often referred to as "psychic sleep." "Usually you are lying down, and often wrapped in a blanket because your body temperature can drop quite a lot when you do it," she explained. "At the most basic, it's a progressive relaxation of your body. It's very relaxing, and it gets you into that state of being physically almost as if you were asleep, but mentally, you're awake—just very, very calm."

One of the key benefits of yoga nidra, according to Dr. Swart Bieber, is that it lets us practice a very particular neurological state. In our normal lives, most of us are either completely asleep or completely awake, running around from the second our eyes open (I'm raising my hand). Even traditional forms of meditation often involve a more active, engaged brain, whether you're being mindful of your breath or repeating a mantra. Yoga nidra is more passive and receptive.

"We're rarely in that middle state of relaxed alertness, where you're not fully asleep, where you're conscious, but you're very, very relaxed," explained Dr. Swart Bieber, who studies and teaches neuroplasticity, the brain's capacity to change over time. One of the benefits of practicing yoga nidra is that because of neuroplasticity, we can essentially rewire our brain to more readily access calmness. Thus, the calm we feel won't only appear in the moments we're doing yoga nidra, but also when we're washing the dishes, walking the dog, or facing a tough task at work.

Small-scale studies have pointed to yoga nidra's ability to increase heart rate variability[1] (a marker of recovery), alleviate symptoms of PTSD, and help with insomnia.[2] I've personally found it helpful in times when I want to feel relaxed in a deeper state than meditation brings me to. Meditation helps me focus; it feels like it calms the buzzing thoughts in my brain, and gives order to my chaotic thoughts. My favorite time to meditate is around 3 p.m., and I use it as a way to get over that afternoon hump and make my mind function for the rest of the day (see page 251 for more on meditation, including why you're likely making it too hard on yourself). Yoga nidra feels like I'm washing out my brain, or tucking it in for a much-needed nap. It feels restorative and restful on the deepest level. I also find it deeply calming—one of my favorite uses for it is on long flights, where it does wonders for combatting my deep-rooted fears of air travel. I also love a Saturday-afternoon session, when I can linger in the relaxation that takes hold, and doing a session before bed, particularly if I need to shake off a stressful day. It's honestly induced the deepest state of relaxation I've felt without drugs, and like Dr. Swart Bieber says, that has carried into the moments that I'm not actively practicing.

You can find yoga nidra classes at many studios, but the easiest way to experiment with a session is to search for free classes on YouTube, Spotify, or an app like Insight Timer (there are literally thousands). Lie down and put a blanket over yourself. Let your body and brain marinate in the sensations and neural connections of true relaxation, and don't be surprised if that sense of calm spills over into the rest of your life.

82.

Take an at-home
silent retreat.

If you've ever wanted a reset without going away and spending a bunch of money or time that you might not have, then this tip is perfect for you. I was interviewing career and business coach Amina AlTai about ways to feel happier and healthier at work when she casually mentioned that she did at-home silent retreats.

I stopped in my tracks. "You do *what*? I need to know more!"

"The majority of people could benefit from a silent retreat," she said. "Perhaps we feel overwhelmed with the state of the world or feel a lot of emotion around us and are unsure what is ours to look at. The moments when we feel we are too stressed to take the time to meditate are the moments we need it most. Getting ahead of those feelings through regular meditation practice and at least an annual silent retreat makes life a whole lot easier."

AlTai says times of transition—such as ending a long relationship, leaving one job for another, or moving into a new home—often create feelings of overwhelm but also offer the opportunity for a fresh start (an idea that science supports; try combining this tip with the fresh start effect on page 20 for even more potent benefits), and serve as perfect moments to get quiet and go deep within. She started her own practice during the COVID-19 pandemic, a time when she was unable to leave the house but wanted to do something that might provide some of the stress-relieving effects of silent retreats she'd done previously. She decided to try a three-day retreat; you can start with any amount of time that makes sense for you.

"One of my favorite teachers once told me to 'start with what you can stand in,'" explained AlTai. "I took that to mean start where you can. Take some time to reflect on what you hope to get out of the retreat, as that may inform how much time you need. One of my meditation teachers once reminded me that 'householders' have different responsibilities than monks that can spend longer durations in retreat. Since we are all living busy lives and are householders, take a look at your schedule and see what is possible for you."

If you want to plan an at-home silent retreat yourself, there are two tips AlTai recommends to make it an easier and more successful experience:

1. **Plan ahead.** You'll want to look at not only your own calendar, but also the calendars of anyone else who closely interacts with your life or depends on you. Make sure that you have no meetings or appointments scheduled; think about what space you'll be in, and if anyone else will need access. What will you eat, and if you have a partner, how will you navigate mealtimes? "If you have kids, a carefully outlined plan with their caregiver for the retreat will be especially important," AlTai said. "Depending on their age, our children may not understand what we're engaging in. If they can understand, having a conversation with them to share what you're about to embark on and your boundaries can be helpful. If they are too young to understand, minimizing your visibility is important. If they can see you but you're not engaging with them, this can cause hurt and confusion. Look for ways to create your own space, or be visibly removed to minimize friction." Make a list of people who need to know about your retreat, and share

what you're doing, and when and how you'll be available. "Nothing interrupts a retreat like a worried call from our mom because we haven't answered a text in three days," said AlTai.

2. **Design the experience.** "Set some intentions or goals for yourself and then ask what would be of service to you and those intentions," said AlTai. "Will you incorporate movement, sound, and breathwork? Decide how many times per day you'll meditate and what practices you'll use." AlTai avoided all screens, and chose two books that she felt would be helpful to her growth to sit with over the three-day period. She also committed to a daily journaling practice. What will the shape of your days look like? What tools will help you achieve the end results you're hoping for?

While everyone will experience different results, according to AlTai, the practice can be transformative. "At the time I did my first at-home silent retreat, the world was in quite a state. I wanted to get clear on my own experience, because heading into the retreat, I felt very reactionary. At the end of my retreat, not only did I feel reenergized, but I was so clear on what my mission was. I felt like I'd dropped an anchor into the earth's center," she said. "Others can expect clarity as well. This is an exercise in detoxing stimuli and everything we take in. What's left is us."

83.

Utilize the healing power of nature.

If you want to restore your attention, relieve pain, or reduce stress, one of the best activities you can do is simply go outside. While light exposure alone offers some amazing benefits (see page 33), spending time outdoors offers myriad rewards.

"One of the most powerful environments that we have available to us for thinking is nature. We live in a world now where we're inside buildings or inside our cars the vast, vast majority of our time, but our species evolved outside," explained acclaimed science writer Annie Murphy Paul. "The kind of information that we find outside in terms of trees, clouds, greenery—all those kinds of stimuli are very easy for our minds to process, and for that reason, it's very soothing and relaxing to spend time outside. The attention we pay when we're outside is different from the kind of attention we have to pay when we're reading little words on a piece of paper or focusing on our screens. The latter is a really hard-edged, intense kind of attention, whereas when we go outside, our attention is drawn here and there in an effortless kind of way."

Psychology professors Rachel and Stephen Kaplan coined the term attention restoration theory to describe the researched replenishing effect time in nature has on our ability to focus. Natural environments help us recover from stress,[1] which then improves our concentration, creativity, and overall feeling of well-being.

Interestingly, the research suggests you don't need to be fully submerged in beautiful nature to reap benefits. "The benefits of attention restoration can come from just taking a walk around your block, even if you live on a city block, or simply looking out the window," said Paul.[2] "I have a big tree that's right outside my own window, and I find myself often just allowing my gaze to soften and my mind to wander as I look at it. The term in the research is known as 'soft fascination.'" In fact, the benefits of attention restoration happen after just forty seconds—yes, *seconds*!—of looking out the window.[3]

"It is a dose-dependent effect," said Paul, "so the more, the better. But if all you have time for is to take a moment to look outside and just let your attention soften that way, that can make a difference in itself."

Beyond its attention-restoring capacities, nature is also a potent stress-reliever. Positive psychologist Dr. Samantha Boardman cited nature as her top antidote to the negative mental health effects of modern life. "One of the most restorative experiences we can create for ourselves is being in nature," she said. "The benefits that it has are unbelievable. Just being outdoors also has this unbelievable ability to interrupt rumination, or that doom scrolling in our mind like, 'Why did I do this? Why did I say that? Why didn't I do this?' Rumination can be an on-ramp to anxiety and depression, and one of the best ways to interrupt it is by being in nature. In some studies, people who are in the middle of a park express the same amount of joy as people on Christmas Day. Studies show that people who are recovering from surgery who have a window into nature require less pain medication. They recover more quickly,"[4] said Dr. Boardman. Even simply sounds of nature played over headphones has been found to increase parasympathetic activation, or our "rest and digest" response.[5]

From a mechanism-of-action perspective, there are a number of things happening. There's the visual elements of nature—the colors, the way the stimuli are distributed—that help create the diffuse attention that Paul mentioned. Beyond that, many plants actually release phytoncides, a type of volatile organic compound that, when inhaled, can reduce blood pressure, enhance immune function, decrease inflammation, and even lead to increases in the quantity and activity of anticancer NK cells.[6] There are also bacteria in nature that have been linked to the release of serotonin.[7] While we're still discovering much of the *why*, and research points to a variety of factors at play in both individual and synergistic ways (the visual stimuli reduce the stress, which reduces your systemic inflammation, which is further impacted by the phytoncides, which further reduce stress, etc.), the evidence is definitive: time in nature is healing both psychologically *and* physiologically, and more time is better.

Look for opportunities to integrate time outside into your schedule. Could you start the day with a circ walk (see page 33) or take a micro walk (see page 52) at various points in your day? Could you catch up with a partner or a friend on a stroll around the block instead of sitting at your kitchen table? Move your desk so you're sitting by a window you can gaze out of?

Beyond that, use nature as a tool when acute issues arise. When you're having a hard time focusing, or you're experiencing a state of stress or pain, remind yourself that research supports you taking a foray into the natural world, however brief it might be. The science is clear—nature heals.

WANT TO DIVE DEEPER?

Listen to this episode of The Liz Moody Podcast:

- "Neuroscience Hacks for Creating Your Dream Life with Dr. Tara Swart Bieber," episode 152

Explore these resources from our expert guests:

- *The Source: The Secrets of the Universe, the Science of the Brain* by Tara Swart Bieber, www.taraswart.com/podcast and @drtaraswart on Instagram

HOW TO
MAKE BETTER
DECISIONS

84.

Practice cognitive off-loading.

One of the best ways to make your brain work better is to get things out of it. "We celebrate people who do things in their heads, like people who remember things without writing them down, or chess grand masters who can plan out many games ahead, all inside their head," explained acclaimed science writer Annie Murphy Paul. "But in fact, the most efficient and effective way to deal with information and ideas is often to get it out of our heads and into physical space." This process, called cognitive off-loading, is critical for both keeping track of things you're trying to store in your brain and also freeing up critical processing capacity.

Post-it notes are one of Paul's favorite ways to practice cognitive off-loading. "You get the benefit of getting all of those ideas out of your head, but then you can actually manipulate those ideas as if they're physical objects, which lets you use embodied resources of being able to physically navigate what is basically a landscape of ideas on the wall," said Paul. "It improves our thinking so much more than if all of the ideas are just locked up in our head and inert. We can get distance from them and dynamically work with them."

I use an app-based workspace for everything from my podcast content schedule to my grocery list to the books I want to read in the future (see the box on the next page for the full list!). It's

A FEW THINGS I COGNITIVELY OFF-LOAD:

- My ongoing grocery list (I add items as soon as I run out of them or think of something I need)

- Recipes I've tried and loved, divided by category (meal prep, breakfast, 15-minute meals, etc.)

- Anything and everything that fills my time (including personal events and goals; see page 145)

- Thoughts or experiences I want to talk about in therapy

- Ideas for podcast topics and guests

- My weekly to-do list

- Future ideas or dreams for my company

- Social media content I want to create

- Media I want to consume later, including movies, TV shows, podcasts, and books

- Places I want to visit, including destinations and restaurants or things to do within specific locations

- Names that I like for potential future kids

- Products or brands that look intriguing (this one actually saves me a ton of money—if I see something I want to buy, I add it to my "Products I Want to Buy" list, which lets me take some time to think about whether the purchase really makes sense, versus the pressure I used to feel to buy something or lose it forever. I get that satisfaction of hitting the "buy" button by simply putting it on my list, and 95 percent of the time, after a few days, I find I didn't actually want the thing, and end up saving money and lessening my waste-stream impact.)

- . . . and so much more—the sky's the limit, so brainstorm and experiment! Try to remove from your brain anything that doesn't absolutely need to be in it.

completely changed my life—I used to think, *Oh, I'll remember that later*, and then I would spend cognitive energy both trying to hold that idea in my brain and then trying to recall it later (and, more often than not, that recall wouldn't work, and the idea would be lost forever).

But more than that, Paul shared, occupying your mind with mundane, memory-based tasks negatively impacts its ability to perform more complicated, and likely more important, activities. "We want to be thinking in terms of freeing up our brains to do what only human brains can do, like imagining, and planning, and creatively putting things together."

If you haven't experimented with cognitive off-loading, give it a try. You can download an app like Notion (my favorite), or use Apple's Notes app, Google Keep, or Annie's physical Post-it trick. Use these tools when you need to physicalize a specific problem to solve it, or more generally to free up the space in your mind for higher-level processing.

85.

Create a failure résumé.

I'm something of a résumé doctor in my friend group. Résumés give us the opportunity to shape our stories in the way we want to tell them. While we might change careers, we can highlight the skill sets that cross over. While we might hate a certain job, we can highlight what we learned and our big wins.

Similarly, creating a failure résumé is a way of shaping the story of your *life* and using the past to create your ideal future. The concept was created by Stanford professor Dr. Tina Seelig, the author of numerous books on personal development. "A failure résumé is a summary of all of your screwups—personal, professional, and academic. You create a line item for each specific transgression, as well as what you learned from it," she shared.

If the practice sounds, well, horrifying, it might be helpful to consider Dr. Seelig's perspective on failure—namely, that it should be free of judgment or shame and, when understood properly, can be used as a tool to transform your future behavior. "Failure is data," Dr. Seelig said. "It is tangible evidence that what you did was incorrect. The act of reflecting on your behavior and the resulting consequences makes the lesson much more tangible and reinforces the insights. You are, therefore, less likely to repeat them. In addition, by writing a failure résumé you are more likely to move on, as opposed to perseverating about mistakes."

Dr. Seelig recommends making a two-column spreadsheet, with

one column for the failure, and one column for what you learned from it.

"Some failures are small and some are monumental. They *all* belong on your failure résumé," Dr. Seelig shared. "A failure résumé is an ongoing document. Our entire life we are learning, and that learning comes from mining failure data to improve. By keeping a mental or physical failure résumé, we acknowledge to ourselves that failure is part of the learning process."

You also don't need to wait for a big failure to get started. "Keeping a failure résumé is a daily act, just like keeping a gratitude journal," Dr. Seelig said. "Each day there are lessons to learn."

At its essence, a failure résumé can help us stop viewing our failures with pain and embarrassment, and instead view them as valuable data. It allows us to gain both distance and clarity from our mistakes, and prevents us from making the same ones again. Start your failure résumé today, and begin to turn regrets into opportunities.

86.

Tap into the intelligence of your body.

If you've ever wondered how, exactly, someone learns to trust their gut, it turns out there's a scientifically backed practice to help you get there. "Our conscious minds are really only a small part of all the mental operations that are going on, because there's so much information that we're taking in as we go through our days that we couldn't possibly be aware of it all," explained acclaimed science writer Annie Murphy Paul. "And yet on some level, our nonconscious minds are taking it in and noting patterns and making connections. Then the question becomes, 'If our nonconscious minds are storing all this information, how do we get access to it?'"

The answer, Paul said, lies in the body: "A little shiver of excitement, your hands getting sweaty. Those physical manifestations are embodiments of what you know on some level deeper than consciousness." That awareness is called interoception, or the ability to tune into our body's physiologic signals, whether it's fullness of the bladder, gut, or bowel, breathlessness, being hot or cold, or feeling our heart beating.

Ignoring those signals is costing us—sometimes literally. "There was a study that looked at financial traders' abilities to sense their hearts beating, which scientists were using as a proxy for general awareness of what's going on inside one's body," explained Paul. The heartbeats were used as a way to measure the traders' interoceptive attunement; while all of us clearly have a beating heart, some of us can tune into the individual beats better or worse than others, which is the "heartbeat awareness" measured in the study. The results were clear: traders who were more aware of their heartbeats were more profitable and more likely to survive in the markets.[1] Essentially, being interoceptive gave traders a measurable fiscal leg up.

If tapping into our interoceptive abilities enhances our performance, the question becomes, how exactly do we do that? The signals are different for everyone—for one person, your "gut" speaking to you might show up as a heavy heartbeat, while for another, it might be tingly hands or a feeling in your stomach. Paul recommends keeping what she calls an interoceptive journal to tune into, track, and identify your unique sensations.

"Make a note of what you're feeling when you're contemplating a certain decision or choice," Paul said. "Then go ahead and make that choice, whether it's picking a stock or making a decision at work. After you've recorded a number of incidents like that, you can go back and see how you felt as you made decisions that you felt, retrospectively, were right or wrong. You'll be able to see how your body has been steering you through these different choices."

It takes time to overwrite what we've been told consciously and subconsciously for, likely, our entire lives—to rely on hard facts and figures, and push through and ignore the more esoteric cues that can't be backed up by data. "But really, these signals carry so much information, so much knowledge, so much experience," said Paul. "To tap into the full potential of our intelligence, we really have to kind of unlearn what society has been teaching us all this time."

Your gut feelings aren't trivial. They're not meant to be ignored in favor of more concrete data. They're valuable information, and learning to tune into them can be a decision-making superpower.

87

Practice decisiveness.

If you find yourself struggling with what to order on a menu, listen up: that lack of decisiveness might be inhibiting your dream life. "What?" you might say. "Calm down. It's just a sandwich. Or maybe a salad? Shoot, I can't decide." But at its core, our ability to be decisive is at the root of our ability to trust ourselves. If you can't trust yourself to choose pastrami over grilled cheese, how will you trust yourself to choose whether to move to a new city, quit your job, or go back to grad school? How will you trust yourself to decide whether you want to have kids or marry your partner? Our lives are *created* by the decisions we make, from the most insignificant to the monumental.

Much indecisiveness also stems from a desire to protect ourselves from discomfort, and practicing decisiveness allows us to teach ourselves that we can *handle the discomfort of choosing wrong.* "When I've tasked people with practicing decisiveness, I've had people come back and share that they experienced so much regret at a meal, because they chose the wrong thing," said renowned psychologist Dr. Aziz Gazipura. "I'll tell them that as bad as that feels, that is your medicine. It is so good for you to learn how to tolerate. Sometimes I get stuff that I love, and sometimes I get stuff that I don't. Maybe now you're stuck in traffic because you picked the wrong way. What's it like to sit in traffic? Are there any hidden gems here? Do you make a phone call to your cousin that you normally don't talk to because now you're sitting in traffic? I help them see that every choice has gifts and things that you don't like."

Every choice has upsides and downsides. How freeing is that? The concept came up again when I talked to Dr. Robert Waldinger, director of the Harvard Study of Adult Development, the world's longest scientific study of happiness. I took our time together as an opportunity to ask him about a question that's long plagued me: whether I should have kids, when, from my outsider perspective, children seemed to make life far more challenging.

"Let's say you don't have kids, and you invest a lot in your work. Then you're going to be more invested in the ups and downs of how your work is going," Dr. Waldinger said. "Life brings us ups and downs. Life brings us challenges. If they're not the challenges of having kids, there are going to be other challenges. If you're alive, you're signing up for a life where challenges come your way."

As humans, we're often guilty of pedestalizing the road not taken. Learning to sit with the discomfort of a confidently selected dinner teaches us that the discomfort isn't inherently *bad*, but rather a part of life. All roads have bumps. The important thing is to *choose* the best path for you, rather than wandering aimlessly or letting someone else dictate your journey.

Dr. Gazipura recommends using small, less significant, and less impactful decisions as a way to build our decisiveness muscle so that in the times that matter, we're more practiced at making both the initial choice and dealing with the positives and pitfalls of the potential result. At a restaurant, skim the menu quickly and go for the first thing that catches your eye. Give yourself ten minutes to research different options for something you want to purchase and then click buy, versus sitting with a million tabs open for months. Pick the first movie or TV show that piques your interest. You'll immediately start experiencing the benefits of less wasted time, more self-satisfaction and self-trust, and greater tolerance for discomfort. And when a bigger decision comes along—Should you reach out to that ex you think might be the love of your life? Should you try a new career path? Should you have kids?—you'll be primed, hands on the steering wheel, ready to turn confidently in the direction of your dreams.

88.

Get specific with
your emotions.

How many times have you said "I'm so stressed"? Hundreds? Thousands, maybe? (I'm raising my hand.) Well, according to Harvard psychologist Dr. Susan David, you might not have been feeling stressed at all—and labeling it as such only makes things worse.

"We use big blanket phrases to describe what we're feeling," she explained. "But think about the world of difference between stress and disappointment, stress and feeling unsupported, stress and that knowing feeling that this relationship isn't working out, or you're in the wrong job or career. If you label everything as 'stress,' your body and your psychology don't have the ability to make sense of that."

The secret to being able to use your emotions in a helpful way is to get specific about what they actually are, and the secret to doing that is to give yourself two other options. The ability to differentiate between your emotions is called emotional granularity, and it has been found in studies to help us better regulate our response to stress[1] and other negative experiences.[2] Individuals with higher emotional granularity experience lower levels of anxiety and depression. They have greater life satisfaction and overall well-being, better social relationships, and a strengthened ability to make decisions. "Sometimes the word 'superpower' is overused, but emotional granularity is literally a superpower," said Dr. David. "It activates what's called the readiness potential in our brains, the part of ourselves that starts to ready us for movement and a pathway forward."

Once you know what you're truly feeling, you can begin to figure out what your next steps should be (if you're having trouble naming more granular emotions, a quick online search for "feelings wheel" will pull up hundreds of options). "I had a colleague who used to describe everything as angry. 'I'm just angry. I'm angry with the organization. I'm angry, and my team is angry.' And I started to say to him, 'What are two other options? What else might you be feeling?' And eventually, he started to say, 'Actually, I'm in a new role. Maybe I'm scared. And maybe my team is not angry. Maybe my team is actually feeling untrusting,'" shared Dr. David. "It's a completely different conversation. This nuance around emotion is very powerful. Yet it's also so simple that you can use it in a meeting or in the midst of a difficult conversation."

The next time you hear yourself say or find yourself thinking: "I'm so stressed" or "I'm just sad," or "he makes me so angry," ask yourself: What are two other options? You'll rewrite your experience in relation to that emotion, and discover more about yourself in that exact moment—and in the long run, you'll begin to access your superpowers.

89.

Have no regrets
when you die.

It's a slogan you see everywhere: "No regrets." But while living regret-free sounds pretty appealing, bestselling author Daniel Pink suggests that it's overhyped. Regrets, he says, aren't necessarily a bad thing.

"Our regrets help us become better decision-makers and better problem-solvers. They help us find meaning in our life," he explained. Research shows that as long as you don't ruminate on your regrets, you can actually find a lot of value in them and they help you gain insights into yourself, among other benefits.[1] "Leaning into our regrets makes us better negotiators, better strategists, and better problem-solvers. If we're doing a problem-solving exercise and then we reflect back and regret what we did wrong, in subsequent exercises, we're going to do a lot better. If we confront it properly, regret is a powerfully transformative emotion."[2]

The problem is that most of us have been taught that regret is shameful, an emotion to be avoided at all costs, which impedes our ability to gain from its myriad benefits. We don't want to ignore our regrets—Pink cites the "No regrets" cliché as a red flag. If you never look backward, or you're not honest in your vision of the past, you'll miss the important lessons embedded in your history.

On the flip side, though, we don't want to wallow in our regrets and let them limit us from feeling the way we want to feel or living the lives we want to live. Like Goldilocks, we're looking for the happy medium, and the good news is, Pink has a specific strategy that he calls "inward, outward, forward." Next time you find yourself grappling with a regret, try the following three-step exercise:

Inward

"Inward is how you frame the regret in the context of yourself," explained Pink. "A lot of times, when we make a mistake and have regrets, we talk to ourselves in cruel and brutal ways. Instead of doing that, we should practice what's called self-compassion, an idea from Dr. Kristin Neff at the University of Texas that encourages you to treat yourself with kindness rather than contempt. Treat yourself as kindly as you treat somebody else. Recognize that your missteps are part of the human condition. This is just a single moment in your life." Be gentle with yourself. Truly internalize the fact that mistakes are an unavoidable part of life and not a failing.

Outward

Next up is outward, which is centered around the concept of disclosure. "Disclosure is a form of sense-making," explained Pink. "Emotions are blobby. They're amorphous." To help turn the blob into something concrete, put it into words. "Words are concrete," Pink said. "Words are less fearsome. That helps us make sense of them."

Disclosure can come in the form of a therapy session, a conversation with someone close to you or even with a stranger (there was a reason people jumped at the chance to participate in Pink's survey!), or a journal entry—as long as you're getting the abstract emotions out of your head and into a more defined—and thus more manageable—form, you've helped make sense of the regret.

Forward

The last step to maximizing the benefits of regret in your life is to look forward. "You *have* to extract a lesson from it," said Pink. "You can't just leave it there. And the way that we extract lessons from our own situation is by getting some distance. It sounds self-evident, but the evidence is overwhelming that we stink at solving our own problems because we're too close to them."

To get that distance, Pink recommended literally talking to yourself in the third person. "Instead of saying, 'What should I do?' say, 'What should Liz do?' It feels silly, but there's a lot of evidence that that's effective,"[3] he said. There are other techniques as well—one that Pink personally likes is pretending you're calling yourself ten years in the future. You in ten years is very much looking out for your best interests. "She knows what you're going to care about. She's gonna be thinking: 'Ten years ago, did I do the right thing? Did I take smart risks? Did I reach out to people I care about? Did I try to establish some stability for my life?' That's what the Liz of the future is going to care about. Give her a call. She'll tell you what to do," Pink said.

Another strategy Pink recommends is making a "New Year's Resolutions, Old Year's Regrets" list. You can do this at the start of a new year, but also the start of a new month or at any life transition. The idea is to add what Pink calls "backward-looking" to the traditional forward-looking goal setting. Ask yourself what your biggest regrets are for the time period you're working with, and then use those regrets to inform the goals you make for the next chunk of time. "If my biggest regret is that this past month, I didn't figure out a way to get time in for exercise, for the next month, I can put exercise sessions on the calendar and make them as sacrosanct as anything that I do," Pink said. Reflecting on your regrets to make the best decisions for current you is a powerful way to figure out exactly how to move forward.

If you're grappling with individual regrets, practice the "inward, outward, forward" structure. If you want to harness your part to supercharge your future, make a "New Year's Resolutions, Old Year's Regrets" list.

Either way, remember: regrets are one of the best tools at your disposal for becoming your best self and living your most authentic, fully-realized life.

WANT TO DIVE DEEPER?

Listen to these episodes of The Liz Moody Podcast:

- "How to Not Have Regrets When You Die with Mega Best-Selling Author Daniel Pink," episode 104
- "What to Do When Things Feel Hopeless: Politics, Climate Change, Chronic Illness, & More with Susan David, PhD," episode 140

Explore these resources from our expert guests:

- *The Power of Regret: How Looking Backward Moves Us Forward* by Daniel Pink, www.danpink.com
- *What I Wish I Knew When I Was 20: A Crash Course on Making Your Place in the World* by Dr. Tina Seelig, www.tinaseelig.com
- *Emotional Agility: Get Unstuck, Embrace Change, and Thrive in Work and Life* by Susan David, PhD, @susandavid_phd on Instagram

HOW TO
BUILD RESILIENCE

90.

Reframe negative emotions.

Fun fact: Your body has a hard time differentiating between certain emotions. "All of our emotions are built from the basic building blocks of our physical sensations," explained acclaimed science writer Annie Murphy Paul. "If you're about to get on a roller coaster, your heart might be pounding, your palms might be sweating. But you might feel those same bodily sensations, but construct them into an entirely different emotion if, say, you're about to give a speech. Your body responds the same way. In both cases, it's preparing you to take on a challenge or a threat."

The power we have, Paul shared, is in how we interpret those bodily sensations. "If we think, 'I'm so nervous, I'm so scared, this is going to be a total flop,' you can get into an anxiety spiral," said Paul. It might sound implausible to reinterpret that sensation as being so excited, but the bodily sensations behind the two are actually the same—and this process, called reframing, is actually far more effective than trying to push those emotions away. "Many of us just say to ourselves, 'Just calm down, it's not a big deal,' but that doesn't work. Your body knows something is going on," Paul said.

Instead, recognizing that you feel those sensations but *attributing* them to a different emotion can radically transform your experience. "Emotion is the thing we construct on top of the bodily sensation," said Paul. You can feel your heart pounding and your palms sweating and think: *Wow, I must be pretty excited about this.*

For reframing to work, the underlying bodily sensations need to be similar—the sensations of excitement, for example, are similar to those of anxiety. The bodily sensations that lead to other emotions map together as well. For example, Paul said, "Sadness can be a very painful emotion, but it also can be very poignant. It can be filled with gratitude, meaning, or nostalgia. If we can steward in the sense of, 'Wow, this thing is so meaningful to me. Maybe it's not in my life anymore, but I really enjoy thinking about it,' as opposed to turning it into something that's dark and negative, it can be really helpful." The bodily sensations might be the same, but the *interpretation* is different, which makes the lived experience entirely different as well.

One of my personal favorite links is between stress and coping. Paul explained: "If we're facing a stressful situation, we can think of it in one of two ways—the very same situation can be either a threat or a challenge. It's a matter of whether we feel that we have the resources to meet that challenge. If we feel that we have the internal and external resources to meet that challenge, then it's activating. It's energizing. It's like: 'I can do this. I can surmount this. I can triumph over this.'"

But, Paul said, if we don't feel like we have the resources, it starts to feel threatening. A helpful way to deal with stress, then, is to turn your attention to the resources that you do have to cope, whether that's knowledge, character, community, or experience. "Thinking in terms of augmenting and highlighting those resources can help you treat a stressor more like a challenge and less like a threat," Paul explained.

The key to this tip? The situations are never changing. Your underlying physiology is still the same: sweaty palms, nausea, a tingling sensation. I'm not asking you to be toxically positive, or to say, "I lost my job, but everything is *amazing*!" That's bullshit. What I'm suggesting is that your brain has the power to change how you interpret those situations. You didn't lose your job because you're worthless; you didn't get a divorce because you're unlovable. How can you interpret it as part of your larger path in life, instead of indicative of the person you are? Similarly, how could you interpret your physiologic signals in a way that's more of use to you? Could your sadness point to a meaning that you could find appreciation for? Could the tightness in your chest be a sign that this really matters to you, and a beautiful reminder that *we get to do things that we feel matter?*

Be a scientist for your own emotions and physiology. The next time you're feeling discomfort, poke around and see if there's an opportunity for reframing. Viewing situations differently is not a trick. It's a powerful neurological tool that yields real-world results.

91.

Create a mental health checklist.

Anxiety and depression have been part of my life for as long as I can remember. In my most severe bout with anxiety, I became agoraphobic, unable to leave my bed without having panic attacks. There were three incidents that I remember vividly from this time: In one, I abandoned my basket in the grocery store line, my rising panic too great for me to wait out the checkout process. Another time my husband asked if I wanted to go watch a rugby game at a local pub with some friends (we were living in London at the time). It was an innocuous social event, one I'd normally accept with an easy yes, but the idea filled me with such surging panic that I couldn't bring myself to go. And last, when, after resigning myself to a life in my bed, I had the thought that if this was it—if every day was going to be this screamingly uncomfortable in my brain and in my body—that life was not, in fact, worth living.

This experience is at the root of my desire to share all the small ways every single one of us can begin to make our lives feel a little bit better moment to moment. But it was also a great lesson in the power of the basics. Since my experience with agoraphobia, people have asked me thousands of times to share the steps that made the biggest difference in my healing journey. And while I've learned so many tiny hacks that have changed my life (many of which I've shared in the book you currently hold in your hands), the thing that truly tipped the scales for my anxiety was stabilizing my foundation.

When I interviewed psychologist Dr. Julie Smith about her favorite mental health hacks, she identified the core components of mental health in a way I'd never heard anyone give voice to before. Before we spend money on supplements, before we optimize that last 2 percent, we need to make sure that we have social connection, good nutrition, routine, sleep, and movement—what she called the five pillars of mental health.

"They're the first things we let slide when we're not doing so well," she shared. "We see them as negotiable—'I'll sleep when I'm done with this project,' or whatever it is. But you take anyone on this earth, no matter how healthy, or strong, or happy they are at the moment, and you start messing around with those five things, and that person will become vulnerable to unhappiness."

To move to England, I left behind my community. There were days when I had no social connection outside of my husband and our roommate, both of whom went to graduate school for long hours. I'd had a full-time job in New York that provided a sharp sense of structure and routine, and while I thought that freelancing would provide a fantasy life, in reality, I was robbing myself of the systems that supported my well-being.

The single greatest choice that truly turned the tide for my mental health was returning to New York, a place where I had community, and getting a full-time job again, which forced my life to again have structure. I suddenly had to wake up early, write a certain number of words a day, and make deadlines. They were all things that intuitively felt like they would *stoke* my anxiety—what if I had a bad night and couldn't sleep in? What if the workload was too much for me to handle?—but in reality, it was exactly what my brain was craving. Structure provides *support*, and my mind was a home that was collapsing in on itself.

Now that I recognize the power of these tools, I don't need them to be place or situation dependent. I can move to new cities, I just need to prioritize maintaining contact with existing relationships virtually, and leaning into local communities in my current location. I work from home, for myself, now, and while I was ter-rified to leave the job that in many ways I credit with saving me, I realized I can create routines that bookend and speckle my day. The *awareness* is the key; after that, it's just a matter of logistics.

To that end, Dr. Smith suggests using the five pillars of mental health as a first line of answers if you're not feeling your best.

I like to keep a list on a sticky note stuck on my computer. I'll find myself catching it out of the corner of my eye and it'll prompt me to do a quick home workout during my lunch hour when I'm feeling a little sad on a Tuesday, or give a friend a call instead of scrolling through social media when I have an interstitial moment to fill. You could even take it a step further and use a habit tracker or a note with checkboxes. Then, instead of playing the guessing game of "Why am I feeling down right now?," you can check the list to help you pinpoint what you might be able to improve.

If you're missing social connection, text or call a friend or fam-ily member. If you've been low on good nutrition, batch cook a big, veggie-packed meal. If your routines have been all over the place—maybe you've been waking up at different times or shirking on the daily practices that make you feel your best—recommit to structure or your favorite habit. We're not going to be able to do everything all the time—there might be a period where you have to work late, or you have a newborn child, or you fall off exercise for a while. The goal, though, is to keep coming back to the list and make sure you're checking off what you can.

"No matter what really complex, amazing therapy techniques you have, if you don't have the foundations there, then it's like try-ing to hold sand in your hands," said Dr. Smith. "It's almost impos-sible. But once you take care of those foundations, you'll be in a much better place to face anything else that comes along."

The five pillars should be your first port in a storm. They are the foundation that you can keep returning to again and again. You only get one body and one mind. They are your home for your journey on this planet; they are far, far too important to build on a shaky foundation.

92.

Remind yourself of your resilience.

You've probably heard of the concept of a gratitude practice—it is, in fact, a core habit of many of the brilliant minds I've interviewed. But have you ever tried a resilience practice? The idea first surfaced when I spoke to renowned death doula Alua Arthur. When I told Arthur I wasn't sure I was strong enough to deal with tough or scary life circumstances, she insisted I was—that we all are.

"When we're doing end-of-life planning sessions, people say things like, 'If I become disabled to a certain point, just take me out back and shoot me.' And I'm like, 'Now, what makes us think that being disabled to that point, we would not adapt to it?' Billions of people adapt to disability all the time. Our capacity grows. Our capacity for grief grows. Our capacity for love grows. We're humans. We're adaptable by nature."

Arthur recommended cultivating a practice to remind us of how resilient we've already been in our lives. "Humans are masters of managing the unknown, because we wake up every day not knowing what it's going to bring us. And yet we adapt to the circumstances. We adapt when our cell phone battery dies and we're in the middle of nowhere. We adapt when we break up. We adapt when we move. We adapt when we change jobs. We adapt when we become parents. We adapt constantly. And we're highly, highly, highly resilient."

If you can acknowledge your past resilience, you'll feel more confident in your ability to be resilient in the future, regardless of what it might hold. Start by writing down a few times you've been resilient in your life. They can be small or significant—maybe you powered through fatigue and stayed late at work to hit a deadline. Maybe you made it through to the other side of a painful breakup. Maybe you endured a difficult medical journey and now are thriving. Maybe you experienced a deep loss and have managed to keep going. Write it all down, and take a moment to really reflect on the resilience that you've *already demonstrated*. Going forward, try to acknowledge and sit in moments of resilience as much as possible. You can face more than you think. You already have.

93.

Make an accomplishments list.

We spend a lot of time counting the things we need to do, and shockingly little time counting the things we *have* done, which can lead to disproportionately negative feelings about the way we spend our time. The reason for this is adaptive and evolutionary: our brains are designed to focus on threats to our survival. Constantly scanning, thinking about future tasks to keep food on the table and lions out of our village was helpful to our ancestors. In the modern world, we're exposed to a million smaller stressors that our brains catalog as threats, while ironically being exposed to far fewer *true* threats to our survival. The result is a high-alert, future-focused brain that's overemphasizing tasks and underemphasizing everything we've accomplished, which can leave us feeling burnt out and like we're on a never-ending treadmill of to-dos.

Productivity expert Chris Bailey has a remedy for that: creating an accomplishments list. "If you feel like you're not making any progress in your life, once a week, write down everything you've accomplished," he said. "If you want, you can break it down by context of your life: your work, your home, your family. You can break it down by the different roles you have: employee, business owner, mother, father, daughter, however you want to think about it. Just write down everything you accomplish. All the milestones you hit, all the projects you finish, all the people you help."

In addition to the weekly accomplishments list, Bailey recommends creating an annual list where you capture ten to twenty things throughout the year that you were able to accomplish.

"It's a wonderful reminder that we're usually more productive than we think we are," he said. "Many of us have productivity dysmorphia, where, similar to how body dysmorphia creates a mental image of ourselves that isn't true to who we are physically, we think we accomplish less than we do. It's worth reflecting on the fact that you might be more productive than you think you are."

Today, create an accomplishments list, and when you accomplish something, write it down (simply lingering in the good feeling of having succeeded at something will literally rewire your neural pathways—you can learn more about that on page 152). Rather than waiting till the end of the week to reflect on the previous seven days, I like to keep a running list on my phone for easy access. When I accomplish something, whether it's turning in a draft of a book, planning a birthday party for Zack, or completing a social media post, I add it to the list. At the end of the week, before I plan my next week (which I do using Bailey's "rule of three"—see page 71), I take a moment to reflect on everything I've accomplished. I also reference my list when feelings of worthlessness seep in—I've even found I get a productivity jolt simply by reflecting on the true productivity I've been able to tap into in the past. If you feel inspired, you can also zoom out a bit and reflect on ten to twenty things you've accomplished over the past year.

We do more than we think. We are more than we think. This is just one little way of reminding ourselves.

94

Use your present relationships to heal your childhood wounds.

We've all heard the old adage about never going to bed angry, right? I've tried for years to adhere to it, which has led to many a sleep-deprived argument that winds long into the night, because conclusions are increasingly hard to reach as your cognitive capacity declines. But my conversation with actor Josh Peck changed my perspective on this practice completely.

"My wife comes from this beautiful, very healthy family system," he shared. "And she taught me that family doesn't leave. So, we can be mad at each other. We can even go to bed angry. But I'll be here and you'll be here when we eventually work this out."

Going to bed angry is a little vote that no matter what state you're in when you fall asleep, the person you love will still be there when you wake up—and that's a powerful message to give them and, perhaps more important, to give yourself. We're *allowed* to have emotions. We're *allowed* to experience the full range of human reactions. The people who love us won't leave us if they see our whole selves.

My childhood ingrained in me the belief that I couldn't rock the boat and still be loved. I had to fit a certain image, play a specific role in the family dynamic—and I've been trying to perform to the best of my ability at the expense of my own well-being ever since.

But one of the most powerful ways we can heal our childhood wounds is through our present relationships—whether they're with close friends or romantic partners. This insight shifted my core belief that true healing is solo work, which further evidences my trauma: We live in a world where relying on others is a necessity for our emotional and physical survival. We're *not* in it alone. To insist on healing in isolation is to disregard that reality. Relational wounds are healed with relational bonds.

Maybe for you, the childhood wound isn't about perfectionism or abandonment, and going to bed angry isn't the specific salve that you need. Maybe for you, it's more about expressing your own needs and desires to a partner, and having that partner validate their importance. Maybe you've had your trust betrayed by childhood figures who broke promises, and you can look to the relationships in your life now to begin to heal that trust.

The first step in this process is to simply recognize those wounds and begin to piece together the ways they might be impacting your life today. Some of us can immediately go back to a resonant experience in childhood—a divorce, a critical or absentee parent, an incident of cheating. If that's you, take a moment to sit in the feelings that come up, and reflect on where those feelings might be poking through today. For others, it might take some digging, either with a therapist or a journal. When I spoke with Vienna Pharaon, a licensed marriage and family therapist and the author of *The Origins of You*, she shared one of the most powerful questions for beginning to identify your childhood wounds: What did you want most as a child and not get?

"It brings us to the pain," she explained. "It brings us to the thing that we craved. I would encourage people to try not to block it. Sometimes I ask that question and they're like, 'I got everything that I needed.' But we exist in imperfect systems. There is no perfect vacuum." Pharaon believes that all of us have some type of childhood pain, and identifying where those wounds are is one of the first steps to healing.

What did you want most as a child and not get? Take a second to reflect on that, and then begin to explore how you can use your relationships of the present to heal your relationship wounds of the past (and no, it doesn't need to be with the same person—Pharaon is adamant that the wound makers don't need to be involved in our healing process). Whether you're simply sharing your wounds with a person close to you (a process called witnessing that Pharaon endorses; we can also witness our own wounds, which is a powerful first step), or beginning to heal those patterns, relying on our current relationships to begin to heal our past ones isn't cheating.

Relational wounds are healed with relational bonds. You're not alone in this world, and your healing needn't be reliant on pretending you are.

95.

Create your own sense of safety and security.

A lot of people these days—myself very much included—struggle with a sense of instability, and the underlying loss of security that accompanies it. For some of us, the world feels fundamentally unsafe in a way that it perhaps hasn't before, and that lack of safety can permeate our everyday psyche. And for others, pervasive systemic failures and structural inequities have long kept the notion of safety out of reach.

While many of the factors that contribute to our sense of stability are out of our control, one thing we *can* do, according to psychologist Dr. Susan David, is become a secure base for *ourselves*. And while that might sound abstract, we can take very practical actions to evoke this sense of inner safety.

"There is literally a five-year-old inside of you that's tapping you on the shoulder saying, 'See me, see me, see me,'" said Dr. David. "What is your five-year-old saying they need? Is it rest, or spontaneity, or connection? What is that child needing from you right now?"

And then, she said, every single one of us has a person inside of us who's fifteen or twenty years older than our current age—so if you're twenty, that person is thirty-five or forty; if you're fifty-five, that person is seventy or seventy-five. "And that older version of yourself is also saying, 'See me. Love me. I need you to be brave. I need you to get some perspective here,'" Dr. David said. "All of us have these very wise people inside of ourselves."

Psychologically, this concept is called continuity of the self. "It's this idea that when we feel stuck, when we feel untethered, we often are very immersed in the experience of that moment," said Dr. David. "But when we start connecting a little bit more in the child part, we can connect more with our feelings and our needs. And in the adult part, we start connecting a little bit more with our values. What does this future orientation of you think of how you spend your time? Who you spend your time with? What would make the adult version of you proud?"

I was raised by two psychologists, and am married to someone who was raised by two psychologists (yes, really). I've spent my life surrounded by the field, and in and out of therapy myself. And yet I've always rebuffed the idea that at the root of so many of my present problems, there was a child self with unmet needs. I wanted to solve my problems in the present, not delve back into my history.

Continuity of self suggests that that childlike part of you is always present—you can simply choose whether to attend to their needs. And if you're not attending to their needs, they'll be apt to do what any child would do when their needs are unmet. They'll cry. They'll act out. They'll get scared. They'll try to protect themselves, and often in unhelpful ways.

I was in my mid-thirties before I stopped trying to "solve" the problem that is my brain and instead asked myself, gently, *What would make the child inside me feel safe right now?* I don't know about you, but for me it's never a logical explanation, rife with statistics and facts. It's never shaming, or berating, or telling that child that they should be over their feelings, that they're having an outsize reaction to reality. I've tried both of those tactics. For years, over and over, I've tried them. And for years, over and over, they haven't worked. Instead, I've learned to tell myself that I'm safe, and I'm loved, exactly as I am. I've even learned to ask people I trust deeply for the same thing. Now when I feel that wavering instability—maybe before a flight, which is a huge anxiety trigger, or maybe because I've learned a piece of scary information—instead of scouring the news to make myself feel better, instead of trying to talk myself into a place of calm, I gently say to myself: *You're safe. You can trust me to keep you safe. You'll be okay.* It might sound floofy, but it works a million times better than any other more rational-seeming technique I've tried.

At the same time, when I feel that lack of stability, I tap into my older, wiser self as well. This works especially well for those more minor things that feel wildly destabilizing—a misunderstanding at work, an argument with a friend, a mistake in a sent email. Tapping into my older self gives me a sense of perspective on the situation, and usually helps me realize how little I'll likely care about this incident in five years (or even five months).

"It's very difficult to read the instructions when you're inside the jar," said Dr. David; this exercise helps you crawl out of those confines and broaden your perspective. Invoking the wisdom of these other versions of you helps you establish yourself as a secure base, allowing you to provide the sense of safety you need to move through the world. There is such power in recognizing that we are both and all: We are the scared children that just want to be told we're safe. We are the wise elders, filled with hard-earned perspective. The next time you're feeling that sense of instability, tap into childhood you. Tap into future you. What do they have to say?

WANT TO DIVE DEEPER?

Listen to these episodes of The Liz Moody Podcast:

- "Mental Health Hacks: Quick Tools for Uncertainty, Loss of Control, Anxiety, Depression & More with Dr. Julie Smith," episode 121

- "Josh Peck on Transcending Childhood Trauma, Hollywood Secrets, Losing 70 Pounds, and Actionable Steps Toward Self Love," episode 103

- "EVERYONE Has Childhood Trauma. Here's Why + How to Heal with Vienna Pharaon, LMFT," episode 164

Explore these resources from our expert guests:

- *Why Has Nobody Told Me This Before?* by Dr. Julie Smith, @drjulie on Instagram
- *Happy People Are Annoying* by Josh Peck, @shuapeck on Instagram
- *The Origins of You: How Breaking Family Patterns Can Liberate the Way We Live and Love* by Vienna Pharaon, @mindfulmft on social media

HOW TO OVERCOME ROADBLOCKS

96.

Get unstuck.

We've all faced moments where we found ourselves stuck, positive that we didn't like where we were but utterly unsure of what to do next. These moments can feel paralyzing, and result in endless rumination about our lack of ability: *I hate my job but I'm not qualified to get another one. I'm not sure I'm with my person, but what if I can't meet someone who's any better? I hate the town I live in, but I don't have the money to move.*

Licensed marriage and family therapist Britt Frank, author of *The Science of Stuck*, has a genius and highly pragmatic prescription for moving through these moments. The key is to start with the assumption that you have three choices in your situation. "They might not be good, but they exist," said Frank. "Even if they're small or crappy choices." Creating consciousness around these choices reminds us of our agency, and that agency begins to create the momentum we need to move through our stuck situation.

Pick a situation where you're feeling stuck—whether it's in your career, your relationships, your environment, or even a behavior pattern you don't like, like reaching for your phone every night or eating food that doesn't make you feel good. Now pretend I told you that you couldn't do anything else until you wrote down three choices for the situation (you can flip through this very book to see some ideas that apply to a variety of situations). They don't need to be the perfect choices; they simply need to be *something* you can do or change.

If truly nothing comes to mind, it might be worth exploring some of the underlying mindsets that keep us stuck. "All behavior, even suboptimal behavior, has a benefit," explained Frank. "Making a change can require fear, unknown, uncertainty, financial risk, relationship changes. It's scary, and it's hard. Even good change requires grief and loss. We have to also ask ourselves honestly, without shaming, 'What am I getting out of not doing the thing I say I want to do?' Name it. Because then you can change it."

Are there any benefits that are keeping you trapped in your current situation? Is there a sense of security that you're afraid to stray from, or a fear of the unknown? Write down the benefits you're experiencing, and then ask yourself: Do they make up for what you're losing? At the end of the day, the choice is yours. What do you want *your* one life to look like?

97.

Fight back against the fairy tale.

Before we even fall in love for the first time, we've received thousands of subliminal messages about what love is *supposed* to look like. In advertising, books, and movies, we're sold over and over the idea of love at first sight, lightning in a bottle. We see princes on white horses and last-minute sprints through airports. It's no wonder that for many of us, what we experience in real relationships is not only not aligned with our expectations, but a disappointment.

According to marriage and family therapist John Kim, that misalignment is actually a *good* thing. "I used to seek out the whole 'walk into a room, meet eyes, the hair on the back of your neck goes up' feeling," he said. "That's what I thought love was. And then I realized that sometimes that lightning in a bottle can be dysfunction. It could be unhealthy patterns from childhood— you may be attracted to this person because it seems familiar and you're used to chaos. Sometimes, if the attraction is that animalistic and crazy, it can be coming from an unhealthy place."

To combat seeking out a spark that could be signifying unhealthy patterns, Kim recommended consciously redefining what you look for in a relationship. "The truth is, love is hard," he said. "People leave their socks on the floor. Living with someone is hard. And so love, to me, is a daily choice. And that choice is: taking ownership, trying to understand before trying to be understood, understanding people's love languages and attachment styles and why they are the way they are, seeing the spirit of who they are, instead of judging them.

"It's really, really hard to do," he said. "Some days are harder than others. But that's what love is. If you glamorize it and think, like, 'Oh, love shouldn't be this hard,' you'll never hit the high notes,' you'll just go through a lot of relationships."

Combatting the outside narratives can be equally—if not *more*—important if you're not currently in a relationship. "A lot of my own anxieties about being single come from society's insistence that happily ever after always means finding your Prince Charming," shared professor of neuroscience and psychology Dr. Wendy Suzuki. "We've heard these stories since we were little."

For Dr. Suzuki, becoming aware of and then questioning the narratives that we've internalized is key. Who said that finding Prince Charming is the only happy ending for a story? "Happily ever after means being as happy as you can be in yourself right now, whether you have a life partner or not," said Dr. Suzuki.

Just because we've been spoon-fed something over and over doesn't automatically make it true; while it may be *a* story, it's not the *only* story. Question which ideals of a "good life" are truly yours and which you might have internalized from years of conscious and subconscious conditioning. This can be a complex process; while a lot of these messages come from the media, everyone around us has internalized that media as well, and can contribute to the cacophony.

Your story is yours to write—not your mom's or dad's, not your best friend's, not advertising executives' or movie producers'. What does your happy ending look like? How can you be the hero of your own journey?

98.

Get to the root of low libido.

One of the most common questions in my DMs is about dealing with low libido, so first, if it's something you struggle with, know that you're definitely not alone. The good news? There are some very straightforward reasons your sex drive might be waning. According to Vanessa Marin, a licensed sex therapist with two decades of experience, there are five factors to consider.

The first is biological. "Are you experiencing any sort of injuries or illnesses, or on any medications that might be impacting your libido? Mental health can fall into this category as well," Marin shared.

Then there's the mental, which Marin said comprises the beliefs we have around sex and the thoughts we have during sex—for example, if you get distracted in the moment during sex because you're thinking of your to-do list, or if you think the man in male-female relationships should always want sex more than the woman.

Then there's the emotional. "Sex obviously stirs up a lot of different emotions for us," Marin said. If you've experienced trauma, you may struggle to stay present in the moment. If you have a lot of shame or guilt around sex, it may be difficult to feel desire for it.

The fourth factor is the relational element. "We often think that our sex life is completely unrelated to the rest of our relationship," shared Xander Marin, Vanessa's husband, who cohosts their podcast and cowrote their book. "But in reality, if you look at the rest of the elements of your relationship—if it feels like the load is imbalanced, if you're resenting things about your partner, if you're always arguing about this topic or that topic—then of course you're not going to feel very much sexual chemistry." He acknowledges that in rare scenarios, people might have incredible sex regardless of how bad things are in the rest of their lives. "But that's the exception, not the rule. The reality is, if you're not feeling very connected in the bedroom, you want to look outside the bedroom. How is everything else in your relationship? And can you work on your connection, your respect for each other, equally sharing responsibilities?"

The fifth foundation is what Marin calls sensual. "That gets into the *quality* of the sex that you're having," she said. "This is another extremely important connection that so few people make. If you're not feeling the desire for sex, ask yourself, 'Is the sex that I'm having *worth* craving?' If you're having sex that feels boring and unpleasurable, if there's nothing in it for you, if it's predictable or routine, why would you crave that?"

You don't need to approach the five factors as homework assignments that you have to complete before you have a higher sex drive. Rather, it's helpful to use them as jumping-off points to explore elements impacting your libido. It's also important to keep in mind that some of these factors might not have easy fixes, or any fixes at all. "It can be really healing for people to say, 'I have this chronic illness that is affecting my libido, and it probably will affect my libido for the rest of my life,'" Marin said. "There can be grief that goes along with that, but I think that acknowledgment is so important."

For the factors that can be addressed, you want to gain awareness of your situation without judgment, and validate what's going on. When you do this, the conversation changes from beating yourself up—*What's wrong with me?*—to recognizing that you've been really stressed at work, or you and your partner have fallen into a pattern of having rote sex that's not stoking your desire that much. From that place of awareness, you're suddenly able to book an appointment with a therapist, or experiment with sex positions or experiences that are more pleasurable.

Having better sex can have huge payoffs both in and out of the bedroom. "One study found that if a couple's sex life is struggling, it takes up eighty percent of their relationship's energy," Marin said. "Conversely, when a couple is in a great place in their sex life, it adds to the relationship. It's this expansive growth."[1]

Outside of its influence on our relationships, struggles with libido can evidence struggles in the life we're living and the choices we're making. "Sex is an opportunity for us to explore ourselves and go deeper into ourselves," Marin said. "Often we write off sex, like, 'You want to have an orgasm.' But it really is an invitation. If you're so busy and stressed and exhausted that sex sounds like the worst possible thing, let's take a look at that. What's going on in your life that you have no time, no energy, no rest, no spaciousness? A prescription like 'Have sex twice a week' is not going to solve that. It's a deeper invitation to ask yourself, 'What's really going on in my life? And is this the kind of life that I want to lead?'"

99.

Reduce your pain.

Have you ever paid attention to what's happening at moments when you feel pain? If your period cramps are especially bad, for instance, have you thought about how much time you've spent outside recently, or how anxious you're feeling? According to Dr. Rachel Zoffness, a psychologist who specializes in pain treatment, understanding these factors and how they influence pain is critical to alleviating it.

"Pain is manufactured in part by your brain's limbic system, which is your emotion center," said Dr. Zoffness. "So if we are not targeting the body, and the brain, and your emotions, and your environment, and all of the things happening inside of you, and around you, we're not actually treating your pain."

Because of that, it's critical to take a biopsychosocial approach to pain, meaning that any pain—from a light headache to chronic pain that leaves a person bedbound—needs to be treated from a biological perspective, a psychological perspective, and a social perspective. These factors contribute to what Zoffness calls a "pain recipe."

"With a baking recipe, you add particular ingredients in a particular order, and bake them in a particular kind of pan at a particular temperature. If you leave out an ingredient, or you bake it at the wrong temperature, or you use the wrong receptacle, you are not going to get the outcome that you want," she explained. "The same is true for pain. There's always a recipe for high pain, and there is always a recipe for low pain. There are biopsychosocial ingredients for everyone that go into a high-pain recipe, whether it's for fibromyalgia or endometriosis, and there is a collection of biopsychosocial ingredients that go into a low-pain recipe."

Dr. Zoffness encourages patients to think about what their last low-pain day looked like and, on the flip side, the constituent parts of their last high-pain day. "For me, with my pain, it's not getting out of bed, or sitting for too many hours in a row," she said. "It's not going outside, or exercising, or moving my body even if it's only for five minutes. It's not connecting with other people and being socially isolated. It's not managing my stress and anxiety, which can pile up. That is my high-pain recipe, and I know that if I have those ingredients in my high-pain recipe, I'm going to have a couple of bad days."

The goal is to fill your days with as many of the low-pain recipe ingredients as possible, and as few of the high-pain recipe ingredients. While Dr. Zoffness has a protocol for doing a deep dive into your personal pain recipe in *The Pain Management Workbook*, I've found enormous benefits in simply paying attention to the ingredients in my personal pain recipes. I've found, for instance, that when I'm physically active in the days leading up to my period—and particularly when that activity takes place outside— I have far more manageable cramps. I've found that I get headaches when I work long hours, when I don't eat meals at regular times or drink enough water, and when my shoulders spend too long hunched around my ears from stress.

It can also be helpful to think of pain as represented by a dial. "A pain dial operates much like the volume knob on your car stereo, and you can turn pain volume up, and you can turn pain volume down," explained Dr. Zoffness. While a lot of different elements impact our pain dials, three things in particular change pain volume all the time: stress and anxiety, mood and emotions, and attention, or what you're focusing on.

"When stress and anxiety are high, your body is tense and tight, your muscles are tense and tight, and your thoughts are worried, your brain sends a message to your pain dial, amplifying pain volume," explained Dr. Zoffness. "The neuroscience shows that pain feels worse when we're in a state of stress and anxiety."[1]

Similarly, when our mood is negative, like when we're depressed or angry, our limbic system, the emotion center in our brain, sends a message to the pain dial, amplifying pain volume. "So pain feels worse when you're having a crap day at work, or you're in a fight with your partner—pain volume is going to be higher," explained Dr. Zoffness.

The third element that always impacts our pain dial is attention, or what we're focusing on. "If you are home in bed, thinking about your pain, ruminating about your pain, focusing on your pain, research says pain volume is going to be higher," said Dr. Zoffness. The good news? "The opposite is also true. When stress and anxiety are low, your body and your muscles are relaxed, and your thoughts are calm, your brain will lower pain volume. When your emotions are positive, you're feeling happy, you're engaged in pleasurable activities, your limbic system will lower pain volume. When you are distracted, you're so absorbed in some activity, you can briefly forget about your pain," said Dr. Zoffness.

Simply understanding the concept of a pain dial and the social and psychological factors affecting pain is enough to change how anyone approaches pain—which is good news, because as Dr. Zoffness reminded us, "None of us, not one of us, is going to escape life without pain."

Playing with the idea of a pain recipe and a pain dial starts to illuminate the many factors at play in the experience of pain, and while not all pain is within our control, it's illuminating and wildly empowering to begin to discover just how much *is*. For any type of pain in your life, start to investigate the ingredients that might make up your high- and low-pain recipes. Explore the different ways you can tune your pain dial and experience the marked benefits of having more control over the pain in your life.

100.

Take the risk.

I get thousands of questions from podcast listeners: "Should I accept a job that requires me to move out of state?" "Should I ask out my friend that I like as more than a friend?" "Should I ask for a raise?" To all of them, I say the same thing: by and large, the science clearly supports you taking the risk.

When I spoke with *The Power of Regret* author Daniel Pink, he described a survey he conducted of 18,000 people from 109 countries around the world. He found that, by and large, people's regrets fell into four categories: foundation regrets, moral regrets, connection regrets, and boldness regrets.

The first category, foundation regrets, "are small decisions that accumulate and become bad consequences over the long run," Pink explained. "They're the regrets of people who spent too much and saved too little. Who didn't take care of their health. There were a lot of regrets about smoking. Foundation regrets sound like, 'If only I'd done the work.'"

Then there were moral regrets. Moral regrets typically involve hurting another person: "I cheated on my spouse," or "I bullied my high school classmate."

Connection regrets are wishing you'd reached out to someone. "They're about the whole spectrum of relationships that we have that end up coming apart," said Pink. "Some of them stick with us, and they stab us with regret. We resist reaching out because we think it's going to feel awkward. It doesn't. And we think the other side is not going to care. They do."

The final category of regrets are boldness regrets, which can be framed as "If only I'd taken the chance." "A lot of people regret not speaking up, not being assertive at work, at school, in their personal life. A lot of people regret not asking people out on dates years ago. People regret not traveling when they had a chance. People regret not starting a business," said Pink. "You can play it safe, or you can take the chance. When people don't take the chance, they've regretted it a lot." Interestingly, when people do take the chance and *it doesn't work out*, they're *still* less regretful than if they hadn't taken it. They know they did everything they could. Time and again, the experts I interview emphasize the same point: we are *far* more resilient than we think. You can deal with the results of your actions. What you can't deal with are the regrets of action not taken.

The best way to avoid boldness regret is to have a bias for action. Switch from asking *what if?*—What if it doesn't work out? What if they don't like me?—to *what now?*, meaning what plan can you put in place to keep the ball rolling? Having a bias for action can even help you figure out what *to* do in the first place. "In any realm, we think that we have to figure out whatever we're doing and *then* do it," Pink said. "But *doing* is a form of figuring out. Having a bias toward action is also having a bias toward figuring things out." Asking someone on a date helps you figure out *how* to ask people on a date and what type of person you'd like to date in the first place. The best way to learn how to write a book is to *write a book*.

To aid in my decision-making even more, I find it helpful to frame the boldness regret in the context of the three other main regrets that Pink found in his survey. If the risk I'm taking pushes me in the direction of reaching out to another person, thus also avoiding a connection regret, that's even more incentive to do it. If the risk, on the other hand, unnecessarily hurts someone's feelings, it might be *creating* a moral regret, an equation that would make me think further about whether it's worth taking. If the risk helps my foundational health, isn't morally negative, *and* enhances my current relationships or builds new ones? Well, that's a slam dunk.

By and large, though, when I find myself asking if I should take a risk, I now lean toward yes, and in the name of avoiding future regrets, I recommend you do the same. Is there an action in your life that you've been holding yourself back from? Take the risk. It might feel scary, but *your* best life is waiting on the other side.

WANT TO DIVE DEEPER?

Listen to these episodes of **The Liz Moody Podcast:**

- "Move Through Trauma, Easily Make Tough Decisions, & Hack Your Vagus Nerve for Instant Calm with Britt Frank," episode 126
- "The Science of Pain: Natural Ways to Manage Chronic & Acute Pain + Hidden Causes with Dr. Rachel Zoffness," episode 141

Explore these resources from our expert guests:

- *The Science of Stuck: Breaking Through Inertia to Find Your Path Forward* by Britt Frank, @brittfrank on Instagram
- *The Pain Management Workbook: Powerful CBT and Mindfulness Skills to Take Control of Pain and Reclaim Your Life* by Dr. Rachel Zoffness, www.zoffness.com, @therealdoczoff on Instagram

Acknowledgments

My last book was called *Healthier Together*, and the concept of community has been a key part of both my work and life philosophy for as long as I can remember. One of my favorite things about writing a book is that it doesn't happen in a vacuum: rather, it's the result of thousands of hours of work by dozens of people. I'm so grateful to all of them—it's unbelievable sometimes that I have so many talented people helping me bring this vision to life.

First—Zack. This book would not exist in this form without you. *I* would not exist in this form without you. You're the most important thing in my life, and the ways that you impact me daily cannot be captured on the page. From shaping the idea for this book to reading the proposal to cheering me on in agent and publisher meetings to combing through every single page for possible edits. This book is riddled with your inputs from cover to cover. Beyond that, you show up in its contents: in the way you've helped me create the bonds that heal my childhood trauma, in the way you help lower my cortisol so I'll live as long as possible (thanks, Dr. Waldinger, for affirming my choice of husband!). You've changed my life in a million ways. I feel lucky every single moment that one day I walked into a bar and found you.

To Ali: Wow. I feel so completely the strength of you being in my corner, and you're such a formidable person to have on my team. Thank you for weighing in, for cheering me on, for advocating for me, for every single thing you've done during every step of this process. I'm well aware that many managers are not invested enough to be texting you in the middle of their South African vacation, and I feel lucky every day that I found someone who I'm so aligned with, who believes so strongly in the work I put into this world.

To Brandi, thank you for never telling me that I'm asking too much, for reassuring me when I felt hopeless, and for always standing up for the book that you knew this could be. I'm so, so proud of where we got, and I thank you for your incredible support on the journey.

To Julie, Emma, Rachel, Karen, Jessica, and Yelena: Thank you for never giving up on this book, or on me. I appreciate you tolerating my perfectionism, and helping me create the book of my absolute dreams. I'm so so proud of what we've made together.

To Jaclyn and Lexi: Thank you for helping this book reach as many people as possible, and being so lovely and fun in the process.

To Gretch!! I love that I finally got to work with you in an official capacity on this book. Thank you for being such a brilliant science writer—I feel extremely fortunate that one of my best friends has a skill set that's so useful to my career! Your willingness to tolerate wild timelines and still do work that surpassed my wildest expectations won't be forgotten. Beyond your literal contribution to these pages, thank you for being such an unfailing support system and the perfect balance of empathy and reason throughout this process.

To Katie, who spent more hours than I can count talking about this book with me. Thank you for being so invested in me, my dreams, and my needs. You support me in all the ways a person can be supported, and you're the kindest human I know. We are sisters by blood but friends by choice and the immense blessing of that is never lost on me.

To my mom and dad, thank you for never telling me my dreams are silly, or dissuading me from taking my non-traditional path. Always having you cheering me on, unequivocally in my corner, has been integral in my success.

To Susan and Leslie. Thanks for being the best second family a person could ask for. Whether you're cheering me on as I push toward a deadline or providing me with conversational relaxation and respite around the table in Berkeley, I feel so supported by you, and I massively appreciate it.

To Jenn! Thank you for being such a critical and helpful part of this book process, and of my company in general. I feel very lucky to have gotten to have you as a member of my team!

To Jenny, Renee, Matt, Logan, Scott, the NYC Book Squad, Justine, Carina, Leigh, Vanessa, Rebecca, Matt, Elizabeth, Tara, and every other member of my unofficial focus group—thank you for weighing in on countless tips, covers and titles, and being so generous with your time and support of me along the way.

To Bella, for the always available cuddles and letting me smell that delicious spot on your neck whenever I needed to. I know you were powering my writing with all of that lap sitting, and I love our little family.

To every amazing guest of *The Liz Moody Podcast*, both featured in this book and not: Thank you for being willing to share your wisdom week after week. I regularly pinch myself that my job consists of getting to ask all of my probing questions to the world's best minds. Thank you for your time, your work, your conversation, and your gifts.

And finally, to the listeners of the *The Liz Moody Podcast* and members of my online communities: I love you. I love that you're so excited to learn and grow; I love that we can laugh together and not take everything so seriously; I love that you support me as much when I'm publishing a book as you do when I'm crying or sharing a moment of anxiety. I get to do this job because of you, and I'm grateful to you every single day for that. Every time I get to talk to one of you in real life or on social, I'm reaffirmed that you're the coolest people around. I love you, and I hope this book ends up well-worn and dog-eared, a reminder of the journey you've taken to create the life of your dreams.

Notes

1. Above all, suffer less.

1. A. Bédard et al., "Can Eating Pleasure Be a Lever for Healthy Eating? A Systematic Scoping Review of Eating Pleasure and Its Links with Dietary Behaviors and Health," *PLoS One* 15(12) (December 21, 2020): e0244292, doi: 10.1371/journal.pone.0244292. PMID: 33347469; PMCID: PMC7751982.
2. M. F. N. Meeran et al., "Pharmacological Properties and Molecular Mechanisms of Thymol: Prospects for Its Therapeutic Potential and Pharmaceutical Development," *Frontiers in Pharmacology* (2017): 8, https://doi.org/10.3389/fphar.2017.00380.
3. A. Gunes-Bayir et al., "Anti-Inflammatory and Antioxidant Effects of Carvacrol on *N*-Methyl-*N*'-Nitro-*N*-Nitrosoguanidine (MNNG) Induced Gastric Carcinogenesis in Wistar Rats," *Nutrients* 14(14) (July 12, 2022): 2848, doi: 10.3390/nu14142848. PMID: 35889805; PMCID: PMC9323991.

4. Figure out your "why."

1. B. A. Dolezal et al., "Interrelationship between Sleep and Exercise: A Systematic Review," *Advances in Preventive Medicine* (2017): 1364387, doi: 10.1155/2017/1364387. Epub March 26, 2017. Erratum in: *Adv Prev Med.* 2017; 2017: 5979510. PMID: 28458924; PMCID: PMC5385214.
2. L. Mandolesi et al., "Effects of Physical Exercise on Cognitive Functioning and Wellbeing: Biological and Psychological Benefits," *Frontiers in Psychology* 9 (April 27, 2018): 509, doi: 10.3389/fpsyg.2018.00509. PMID: 29755380; PMCID: PMC5934999.
3. M. C. Pascoe et al., "Single Session and Short-Term Exercise for Mental Health Promotion in Tertiary Students: A Scoping Review," *Sports Medicine - Open* 7(1) (October 11, 2021): 72, doi: 10.1186/s40798-021-00358-y. PMID: 34635969; PMCID: PMC8505587.
4. Stephen Bruehl, "Are Endogenous Opioid Mechanisms Involved in the Effects of Aerobic Exercise Training on Chronic Low Back Pain: A Randomized Controlled Trial," *Pain* (December 2020), https://journals.lww.com/pain/Citation/2020/12000/Are_endogenous_opioid_mechanisms_involved_in_the.23.aspx.
5. G. Prabu Raja et al., "Effectiveness of Deep Cervical Fascial Manipulation and Yoga Postures on Pain, Function, and Oculomotor Control in Patients with Mechanical Neck Pain: Study Protocol of a Pragmatic, Parallel-Group, Randomized, Controlled Trial," *Trials* 22, no. 1 (August 28, 2021): 1–14, https://doi.org/10.1186/s13063-021-05533-w.
6. M. Shohani et al., "The Effect of Yoga on Stress, Anxiety, and Depression in

Women," *International Journal of Preventive Medicine* 9(21) (February 2018), doi: 10.4103/ijpvm.IJPVM_242_16. PMID: 29541436; PMCID: PMC5843960.

7.   S. Ranabir and K. Reetu, "Stress and Hormones," *Indian Journal of Endocrinology and Metabolism* 15(1) (January 2011): 18–22, doi: 10.4103/2230-82 10.77573. PMID: 21584161; PMCID: PMC3079864.

5. Utilize the fresh start effect.

1.   Hengchen Dai, Katherine L. Milkman, and Jason Riis, "The Fresh Start Effect: Temporal Landmarks Motivate Aspirational Behavior," *Management Science* 60, no. 10 (October 2014): 2563–82, https://doi.org/10.1287/mnsc.2014.1901.

7. Use a success framework.

1.   L. B. Pham and S. E. Taylor, "From Thought to Action: Effects of Process-versus Outcome-Based Mental Simulations on Performance," *Personality and Social Psychology Bulletin* 25(2): 250–60, https://doi.org/10.1177/01461672990250 02010.

2.   Gabriele Oettingen et al., "Self-Regulation of Time Management: Mental Contrasting with Implementation Intentions," *European Journal of Social Psychology* 45, no. 2 (March 2015): 218–29, https://doi.org/10.1002/ejsp.2090; Andreas Kappes, Henrik Singmann, and Gabriele Oettingen, "Mental Contrasting Instigates Goal Pursuit by Linking Obstacles of Reality with Instrumental Behavior," *Journal of Experimental Social Psychology* 48, no. 4 (July 2012): 811–18, https://doi.org/10.1016/j.jesp.2012.02.002.

3.   G. Stadler, G. Oettingen, and P. M. Gollwitzer, "Physical Activity in Women: Effects of a Self-regulation Intervention," *American Journal of Preventive Medicine* 36(1) (2009): 29–34, doi:10.1016/j.amepre.2008.09.021.

4.   M. A. Adriaanse, D. T. De Ridder, and I. Voorneman, "Improving Diabetes Self-management by Mental Contrasting," *Psychology and Health* 28(1) (2013): 1–12, doi: 10.1080/08870446.2012.660154

5.   D. Saddawi-Konefka et al., "Changing Resident Physician Studying Behaviors: A Randomized, Comparative Effectiveness Trial of Goal Setting Versus Use of WOOP," *Journal of Graduate Medical Education* 9(4) (2017): 451–57, doi:10.4300/JGME-D-16-00703.1.

6.   Nora Rebekka Krott and Gabriele Oettingen, "Mental Contrasting of Counterfactual Fantasies Attenuates Disappointment, Regret, and Resentment," *Motivation and Emotion* 42, no. 1 (October 31, 2017): 17–36, https://doi.org /10.1007/s11031-017-9644-4.

7.   Gabriele Oettingen et al., "Self-Regulation of Time Management: Mental Contrasting with Implementation Intentions," *European Journal of Social Psychology* 45, no. 2 (March 2015): 218–29, https://doi.org/10.1002/ejsp .2090.

8. Try temptation bundling.

1.   Katherine L. Milkman, Julia A. Minson, and Kevin G. M. Volpp, "Holding the Hunger Games Hostage at the Gym: An Evaluation of Temptation Bundling," *Management Science* 60, no. 2 (February 1, 2014), https://doi.org/10.1287 /mnsc.2013.1784.

9. Take a circ walk.

1.   Ngoc-Hien Du and Steven A Brown, "Measuring Circadian Rhythms in Human Cells – PubMed," *Methods in Molecular Biology* 2130 (January 1, 2021), https://doi.org/10.1007/978-1-0716-0381-9_4.

2. Melinda A. Ma and Elizabeth H. Morrison, "Neuroanatomy, Nucleus Supra-chiasmatic," *NCBI Bookshelf*, July 25, 2022, https://www.ncbi.nlm.nih.gov/books/NBK546664/.
3. Ellen R. Stothard et al., "Circadian Entrainment to the Natural Light-Dark Cycle across Seasons and the Weekend," *Current Biology* 27, no. 4 (February 20, 2017): 508–13, https://doi.org/10.1016/j.cub.2016.12.041.

11. Identify your chronotype.

1. Ángel Correa et al., "Circadian Rhythms and Decision-Making: A Review and New Evidence from Electroencephalography – PubMed," *Chronobiology International* 37, no. 4 (April 1, 2020), https://doi.org/10.1080/07420528.2020.1715421.
2. R. G. Foster, "Fundamentals of Circadian Entrainment by Light," *Lighting Research & Technology* 53, no. 5 (July 20, 2021): 377–93, https://doi.org/10.1177/14771535211014792.
3. McGlashan Cain et al., "Evening Home Lighting Adversely Impacts the Circadian System and Sleep," *Scientific Reports* 10, no. 1 (November 5, 2020): 1–10, https://doi.org/10.1038/s41598-020-75622-4.
4. Katya Kovac et al., "Exercising Caution Upon Waking–Can Exercise Reduce Sleep Inertia?," *Frontiers in Physiology* 11 (April 7, 2020), https://doi.org/10.3389/fphys.2020.00254.

13. Create metabolically optimized meals.

1. Miguel A. Sanchez-Garrido and Manuel Tena-Sempere, "Metabolic Dysfunction in Polycystic Ovary Syndrome: Pathogenic Role of Androgen Excess and Potential Therapeutic Strategies," *Molecular Metabolism* 35 (May 1, 2020), https://doi.org/10.1016/j.molmet.2020.01.001.
2. J. A. Dunbar et al., "Depression: An Important Comorbidity with Metabolic Syndrome in a General Population," *Diabetes Care* 31(12) (December 2008): 2368–73, doi: 10.2337/dc08-0175. Epub October 3, 2008. PMID: 18835951; PMCID: PMC2584197.
3. N. J. Goodson et al., "Cardiovascular Risk Factors Associated with the Metabolic Syndrome Are More Prevalent in People Reporting Chronic Pain: Results from a Cross-sectional General Population Study," *Pain* 154(9) (2013): 1595–1602, doi:10.1016/j.pain.2013.04.043.
4. NHLBI, NIH, "What Is Metabolic Syndrome?," n.d., https://www.nhlbi.nih.gov/health/metabolic-syndrome.
5. R. Westerman and A. K. Kuhnt, "Metabolic Risk Factors and Fertility Disorders: A Narrative Review of the Female Perspective," *Reproductive Biomedecine & Society Online* 14 (October 1, 2021): 66–74, doi: 10.1016/j.rbms.2021.09.002. PMID: 34765754; PMCID: PMC8569630.
6. E. Sanchez, A. W. Pastuszak, and M. Khera, "Erectile Dysfunction, Metabolic Syndrome, and Cardiovascular Risks: Facts and Controversies," *Translational Andrologu and Urology* 6(1) (February 2017): 28–36, doi: 10.21037/tau.2016.10.01. PMID: 28217448; PMCID: PMC5313297.
7. R. K. Naviaux et al., "Metabolic Features of Chronic Fatigue Syndrome," *Proceedings of the National Academy of Sciences* 113(37) (2016), https://doi.org/10.1073/pnas.1607571113.
8. Meghan O'Hearn et al., "Trends and Disparities in Cardiometabolic Health Among U.S. Adults, 1999-2018," *Journal of the American College of Cardiology* 80, no. 2 (July 12, 2022): 138–51, https://doi.org/10.1016/j.jacc.2022.04.046.

9. K. E. Lane et al., "Bioavailability and Conversion of Plant Based Sources of Omega-3 Fatty Acids: A Scoping Review to Update Supplementation Options for Vegetarians and Vegans," *Critical Reviews in Food Science and Nutrition* 62(18) (2022): 4982–97, doi:10.1080/10408398.2021.1880364.

14. Do micro-workouts for mega-benefits.

1. Michael Holmstrup et al., "Multiple Short Bouts of Exercise over 12-h Period Reduce Glucose Excursions More than an Energy-Matched Single Bout of Exercise," *Metabolism: Clinical and Experimental* 63, no. 4 (April 2014): 510–19, https://doi.org/10.1016/j.metabol.2013.12.006.
2. Jung Ha Park et al., "Sedentary Lifestyle: Overview of Updated Evidence of Potential Health Risks," *Korean Journal of Family Medicine* 41, no. 6 (November 1, 2020), https://doi.org/10.4082/kjfm.20.0165.

16. Activate your body's natural glucose sponges.

1. L. Mayans, "Metabolic Syndrome: Insulin Resistance and Prediabetes," *FP Essentials* 435 (2015): 11–16.
2. S. Moreno-Fernández et al., "High Fat/High Glucose Diet Induces Metabolic Syndrome in an Experimental Rat Model," *Nutrients* 10(10) (October 14, 2018): 1502, doi: 10.3390/nu10101502. PMID: 30322196; PMCID: PMC621 3024.
3. Aidan J. Buffey et al., "The Acute Effects of Interrupting Prolonged Sitting Time in Adults with Standing and Light-Intensity Walking on Biomarkers of Cardiometabolic Health in Adults: A Systematic Review and Meta-Analysis," *Sports Medicine* 52, no. 8 (February 11, 2022): 1765–87, https://doi.org/10.1007/s40279-022-01649-4.

18. Take a cold shower.

1. Jonathan D. C. Leeder et al., "Cold Water Immersion Improves Recovery of Sprint Speed Following a Simulated Tournament," *European Journal of Sport Science* 19, no. 9 (October 1, 2019), https://doi.org/10.1080/17461391.2019.1 585478.
2. Denis Blondin et al., "Increased Brown Adipose Tissue Oxidative Capacity in Cold-Acclimated Humans," *Journal of Clinical Endocrinology & Metabolism* 99, no. 3 (March 1, 2014): E438–46, https://doi.org/10.1210/jc.2013-3901.
3. J. Leppäluoto et al., "Effects of Long-Term Whole-Body Cold Exposures on Plasma Concentrations of ACTH, Beta-Endorphin, Cortisol, Catecholamines and Cytokines in Healthy Females," *Scandinavian Journal of Clinical and Laboratory Investigation* 68, no. 2 (January 2008): 145–53, https://doi.org/10.1080/00365510701516350.
4. D. G. Johnson et al., "Plasma Norepinephrine Responses of Man in Cold Water – PubMed," *Journal of Applied Physiology: Respiratory, Environmental and Exercise Physiology* 43, no. 2 (August 1, 1977), https://doi.org/10.1152/jappl.1977.43.2.216.
5. Nikolai A. Shevchuk, "Adapted Cold Shower as a Potential Treatment for Depression – PubMed," *Medical Hypotheses* 70, no. 5 (January 1, 2008), https://doi.org/10.1016/j.mehy.2007.04.052.
6. G. A. Buijze et al., "The Effect of Cold Showering on Health and Work: A Randomized Controlled Trial," *PLoS One* 11(9) (September 15, 2016): e016174, doi: 10.1371/journal.pone.0161749. Erratum in: *PLoS One* 13(8) (August 2, 2018): e0201978. PMID: 27631616; PMCID: PMC5025014.

22. Overcome procrastination.

1. Todd Rogers, "Commitment Devices: Using Initiatives to Change Behavior," *JAMA* 311, no. 20 (May 28, 2014): 2065–66, https://doi.org/10.1001/jama.2014.3485.
2. B. B. Gump and K. A. Matthews, "Are Vacations Good for Your Health? The 9-Year Mortality Experience after the Multiple Risk Factor Intervention Trial—PubMed," *Psychosomatic Medicine* 62, no. 5 (October 1, 2000), https://doi.org/10.1097/00006842-200009000-00003.
3. "Glassdoor Survey Finds Americans Forfeit Half of Their Earned Vacation/Paid Time Off," Glassdoor About Us, May 24, 2017, https://www.glassdoor.com/about-us/glassdoor-survey-finds-americans-forfeit-earned-vacationpaid-time/.

23. Artificially limit your time.

1. Day Week Global, "The Results Are In: The UK's Four-Day Week Pilot," *Autonomy*, February 2023.

26. Gesture and fidget more.

1. Jennie E. Pyers et al., "Gesture Helps, Only If You Need It: Inhibiting Gesture Reduces Tip-of-the-Tongue Resolution for Those with Weak Short-Term Memory," *Cognitive Science* 45, no. 1 (January 2021): e12914, https://doi.org/10.1111/cogs.12914.
2. Susan Wagner Cook, Terina KuangYi Yip, and Susan Goldin-Meadow, "Gesturing Makes Memories That Last," *Journal of Memory and Language* 63, no. 4 (November 2010): 465–75, https://doi.org/10.1016/j.jml.2010.07.002.

27. Do nothing (with intention).

1. Niyat Henok, Frédéric Vallée-Tourangeau, and Gaëlle Vallée-Tourangeau, "Incubation and Interactivity in Insight Problem Solving," *Psychological Research* 84, no. 1 (February 2020): 128–39, https://doi.org/10.1007/s00426-018-0992-9.

34. Overcome impostor syndrome.

1. Dena M. Bravata et al., "Commentary: Prevalence, Predictors, and Treatment of Imposter Syndrome: A Systematic Review," *Journal of Mental Health & Clinical Psychology* 4, no. 3 (August 24, 2020).

40. Build belief in yourself.

1. Bill Taylor, "What Breaking the 4-Minute Mile Taught Us about the Limits of Conventional Thinking," *Harvard Business Review*, March 9, 2018, https://hbr.org/2018/03/what-breaking-the-4-minute-mile-taught-us-about-the-limits-of-conventional-thinking.

44. Build tolerance for hard things.

1. Rafael Franco, Irene Reyes-Resina, and Gemma Navarro, "Dopamine in Health and Disease: Much More Than a Neurotransmitter," *Biomedicines* 9, no. 2 (February 1, 2021), https://doi.org/10.3390/biomedicines9020109.

45. Rewire your neural pathways for happiness.

1. Rick Hanson et al., "Learning to Learn from Positive Experiences," *Journal of Positive Psychology* 18, no. 1 (2021): 142–53, https://doi.org/10.1080/17439760.2021.2006759.

46. Do something for someone else.

1. Cassie Mogilner, Zoë Chance, and Michael I. Norton, "Giving Time Gives You Time," *Psychological Science* 23, no. 10 (September 12, 2012): 1233–38, https://doi.org/10.1177/0956797612442551.

2. Rebecca E. Cooney et al., "Neural Correlates of Rumination in Depression," *Cognitive, Affective & Behavioral Neuroscience* 10(4) (December 2010): 470–78, https://doi.org/10.3758/CABN.10.4.470.

47. Fill your life with joy.

1. Y. Iwasaki et al., "Voices from the Margins: Stress, Active Living, and Leisure as a Contributor to Coping with Stress," *Leisure Sciences* 28 (2006): 163–80.

2. K. Tominaga et al., "Family Environment, Hobbies and Habits as Psychosocial Predictors of Survival for Surgically Treated Patients with Breast Cancer," *Japanese Journal of Clinical Oncology* 28(1) (1998): 36–41, doi:10.1093/jjco/28.1.36.

3. J. S. House, K. R. Landis, and D. Umberson, "Social Relationships and Health," *Science* 241(4865) (1988): 540–45, doi:10.1126/science.3399889.

50. Take advantage of the mere exposure effect.

1. Richard L. Moreland and Scott R. Beach, "Exposure Effects in the Classroom: The Development of Affinity among Students," *Journal of Experimental Social Psychology* 28, no. 3 (May 1992): 255–76, https://doi.org/10.1016/0022-1031(92)90055-O.

53. Become a winning conversationalist.

1. Alison Wood Brooks and Francesca Gino, "It Doesn't Hurt to Ask: Question-Asking Increases Liking," Harvard Business School, September 2017, https://www.hbs.edu/faculty/Pages/item.aspx?num=52115.

54. Deepen your existing friendships.

1. Robert Waldinger, MD, and Marc Schulz, PhD, *The Good Life: Lessons from the World's Longest Scientific Study of Happiness* (New York: Simon and Schuster, 2023).

2. N. L. Collins and L. C. Miller, "Self-Disclosure and Liking: A Meta-Analytic Review," *Psychological Bulletin* 116, no. 3 (November 1, 1994), https://doi.org/10.1037/0033-2909.116.3.457.

57. Take your sex life to the next level.

1. Yangmei Luo et al., "Well-Being and Anticipation for Future Positive Events: Evidences from an fMRI Study," *Frontiers in Psychology* 8 (January 9, 2018), https://doi.org/10.3389/fpsyg.2017.02199.

2. Samantha A. Wagner et al., "Touch Me Just Enough: The Intersection of Adult Attachment, Intimate Touch, and Marital Satisfaction," *Journal of Social and Personal Relationships* 37, no. 6 (March 25, 2020): 1945–67, https://doi.org/10.1177/0265407520910791.

3. Beate Ditzen, Christiane Hoppmann, and Petra Klumb, "Positive Couple Interactions and Daily Cortisol: On the Stress-Protecting Role of Intimacy," *Psychosomatic Medicine* 70, no. 8 (October 1, 2008), https://doi.org/10.1097/PSY.0b013e318185c4fc.

4. Kerstin Uvnas-Moberg and Maria Petersson, "[Oxytocin, a Mediator of Anti-Stress, Well-Being, Social Interaction, Growth and Healing]," *Zeitschrift Fur Psychosomatische Medizin Und Psychotherapie* 51, no. 1 (January 1, 2005), https://doi.org/10.13109/zptm.2005.51.1.57.

59. Eat thirty types of plants per week.

1. Daniel McDonald et al., "American Gut: An Open Platform for Citizen Science Microbiome Research," *mSystems* 3, no. 3 (June 1, 2018), https://doi.org/10.1128/mSystems.00031-18.

2. S. N. Bhupathiraju and K. L. Tucker, "Greater Variety in Fruit and Vegetable Intake Is Associated with Lower Inflammation in Puerto Rican Adults," *American Journal of Clinical Nutrition* 93(1) (2011): 37–46, doi:10.3945/ajcn.2010.29913.

3. G. Turner-McGrievy and M. Harris, "Key Elements of Plant-based Diets Associated with Reduced Risk of Metabolic Syndrome," *Current Diabetes Reports* 14(9) (2014): 524, doi:10.1007/s11892-014-0524-y.

4. A. Janet Tomiyama et al., "Low Calorie Dieting Increases Cortisol," *Psychosomatic Medicine* 72, no. 4 (May 2010): 357–64, https://doi.org/10.1097/PSY.0b013e3181d9523c.

5. C. E. Howard and L. K. Porzelius, "The Role of Dieting in Binge Eating Disorder: Etiology and Treatment Implications," *Clinical Psychology Review* 19, no. 1 (January 1, 1999), https://doi.org/10.1016/s0272-7358(98)00009-9.

6. J. Menzel et al., "Systematic review and meta-analysis of the associations of vegan and vegetarian diets with inflammatory biomarkers," *Scientific Reports* 10(1) (December 10, 2020): 21736, doi: 10.1038/s41598-020-78426-8. PMID: 33303765; PMCID: PMC7730154.

7. H. Kim, L. E. Caulfield, and C. M. Rebholz, "Healthy Plant-Based Diets Are Associated with Lower Risk of All-Cause Mortality in US Adults," *Journal of Nutrition* 148(4) (April 1, 2018): 624–31, doi: 10.1093/jn/nxy019. PMID: 29659968; PMCID: PMC6669955.

8. J. Alcock, C. C. Maley, and C. A. Aktipis, "Is Eating Behavior Manipulated by the Gastrointestinal Microbiota? Evolutionary Pressures and Potential Mechanisms," *Bioessays* 36(10) (October 2014): 940–49, doi: 10.1002/bies.201400071. Epub August 8, 2014. PMID: 25103109; PMCID: PMC4270213.

60. Cook and cool your carbs.

1. Karolina Kaźmierczak-Siedlecka et al., "Sodium Butyrate in Both Prevention and Supportive Treatment of Colorectal Cancer," *Frontiers in Cellular and Infection Microbiology* 12 (October 26, 2022), https://doi.org/10.3389/fcimb.2022.1023806.

2. Celeste Alexander et al., "Perspective: Physiologic Importance of Short-Chain Fatty Acids from Nondigestible Carbohydrate Fermentation," *Advances in Nutrition* 10, no. 4 (July 1, 2019), https://doi.org/10.1093/advances/nmz004.

3. Jin He et al., "Short-Chain Fatty Acids and Their Association with Signalling Pathways in Inflammation, Glucose and Lipid Metabolism," *International Journal of Molecular Sciences* 21, no. 17 (September 1, 2020), https://doi.org/10.3390/ijms21176356.

4. Diane F. Birt et al., "Resistant Starch: Promise for Improving Human Health," *Advances in Nutrition* 4, no. 6 (November 1, 2013), https://doi.org/10.3945/an.113.004325.

5. A. P. Nugent, "Health Properties of Resistant Starch," *Nutrition Bulletin* 30, no. 1 (February 16, 2005): 27–54, https://doi.org/10.1111/j.1467-3010.2005.00481.x.

6. Shujun Wang et al., "Starch Retrogradation: A Comprehensive Review," *Comprehensive Reviews in Food Science and Food Safety* 14, no. 5 (July 14, 2015): 568–85, https://doi.org/10.1111/1541-4337.12143.

61. Incorporate more fermented foods.

1. Yangmei Luo et al., "Well-Being and Anticipation for Future Positive Events: Evidences from an fMRI Study," *Frontiers in Psychology* 8 (January 9, 2018), https://doi.org/10.3389/fpsyg.2017.02199.
2. Hannah C. Wastyk et al., "Gut-Microbiota-Targeted Diets Modulate Human Immune Status," *Cell* 184, no. 16 (August 5, 2021): 4137–53.e14, https://doi.org/10.1016/j.cell.2021.06.019.
3. Hannah C. Wastyk et al., "Gut-Microbiota-Targeted Diets Modulate Human Immune Status," *Cell* 184, no. 16 (August 5, 2021): 4137–53.e14, https://doi.org/10.1016/j.cell.2021.06.019.

62. Get dirty.

1. D. P. Strachan, "Hay Fever, Hygiene, and Household Size," *BMJ (Clinical Research Ed.)* 299, no. 6710 (November 18, 1989): 1259–60, https://doi.org/10.1136/bmj.299.6710.1259.
2. Marina D. Brown et al., "Fecal and Soil Microbiota Composition of Gardening and Non-Gardening Families," *Scientific Reports* 12, no. 1 (January 31, 2022): 1–12, https://doi.org/10.1038/s41598-022-05387-5.
3. Min Zhao et al., "Beneficial Associations of Low and Large Doses of Leisure Time Physical Activity with All-Cause, Cardiovascular Disease and Cancer Mortality: A National Cohort Study of 88,140 US Adults," *British Journal of Sports Medicine* 53, no. 22 (November 1, 2019): 1405–11, https://doi.org/10.1136/bjsports-2018-099254.

63. Don't unnecessarily eliminate foods.

1. Peter C. Konturek, T. Brzozowski, and S. J. Konturek, "Stress and the Gut: Pathophysiology, Clinical Consequences, Diagnostic Approach and Treatment Options – PubMed," *Journal of Physiology and Pharmacology : An Official Journal of the Polish Physiological Society* 62, no. 6 (December 1, 2011).
2. Giada De Palma et al., "Effects of a Gluten-Free Diet on Gut Microbiota and Immune Function in Healthy Adult Human Subjects," *British Journal of Nutrition* 102, no. 8 (October 1, 2009), https://doi.org/10.1017/S0007114509371767; Angela Genoni et al., "Long-Term Paleolithic Diet Is Associated with Lower Resistant Starch Intake, Different Gut Microbiota Composition and Increased Serum TMAO Concentrations," *European Journal of Nutrition* 59, no. 5 (August 2020): 1845–58, https://doi.org/10.1007/s00394-019-02036-y.

64. Feed your good gut bacteria.

1. Jakub Żółkiewicz et al., "Postbiotics—A Step Beyond Pre- and Probiotics," *Nutrients* 12, no. 8 (July 23, 2020): 2189, https://doi.org/10.3390/nu12082189.
2. Jian Tan et al., "The Role of Short-Chain Fatty Acids in Health and Disease – PubMed," *Advances in Immunology* 121 (January 1, 2014), https://doi.org/10.1016/B978-0-12-800100-4.00003-9.
3. Camille Danne and Harry Sokol, "Butyrate, a New Microbiota-Dependent Player in CD8+ T Cells Immunity and Cancer Therapy?," *Cell Reports Medicine* 2, no. 7 (July 20, 2021), https://doi.org/10.1016/j.xcrm.2021.100328.
4. Christine N. Spencer et al., "Dietary Fiber and Probiotics Influence the Gut Microbiome and Melanoma Immunotherapy Response," *Science* 374, no. 6575 (December 24, 2021), https://doi.org/10.1126/science.aaz7015.
5. Mingyang Song et al., "Fiber Intake and Survival after Colorectal Cancer Diagnosis," *JAMA Oncology* 4, no. 1 (January 1, 2018), https://doi.org/10.1001/jamaoncol.2017.3684.

65. Eliminate bloating and constipation.

1. Doris Vandeputte et al., "Stool Consistency Is Strongly Associated with Gut Microbiota Richness and Composition, Enterotypes and Bacterial Growth Rates," *Gut* 65, no. 1 (June 11, 2015): 57–62, https://doi.org/10.1136/gutjnl -2015-309618; Francesco Asnicar et al., "Blue Poo: Impact of Gut Transit Time on the Gut Microbiome Using a Novel Marker," *Gut* 70, no. 9 (September 2021): 1665–74, https://doi.org/10.1136/gutjnl-2020-323877.

66. Reframe stress relief.

1. Viktoriya Maydych, "The Interplay Between Stress, Inflammation, and Emotional Attention: Relevance for Depression," *Frontiers in Neuroscience* 13 (January 1, 2019), https://doi.org/10.3389/fnins.2019.00384.
2. Karen Bohmwald et al., "Contribution of Cytokines to Tissue Damage During Human Respiratory Syncytial Virus Infection," *Frontiers in Immunology* 10 (January 1, 2019), https://doi.org/10.3389/fimmu.2019.00452.
3. Manfred G. Kitzbichler et al., "Peripheral Inflammation Is Associated with Micro-Structural and Functional Connectivity Changes in Depression-Related Brain Networks," *Molecular Psychiatry* 26, no. 12 (September 17, 2021): 7346–54, https://doi.org/10.1038/s41380-021-01272-1.
4. Lihua Duan, Xiaoquan Rao, and Keshav Raj Sigdel, "Regulation of Inflammation in Autoimmune Disease," *Journal of Immunology Research* (January 1, 2019), https://doi.org/10.1155/2019/7403796.
5. Daniela Sorriento and Guido Iaccarino, "Inflammation and Cardiovascular Diseases: The Most Recent Findings," *International Journal of Molecular Sciences* 20, no. 16 (August 1, 2019), https://doi.org/10.3390/ijms20163879.
6. Theoharis C. Theoharides et al., "Brain 'Fog,' Inflammation and Obesity: Key Aspects of Neuropsychiatric Disorders Improved by Luteolin," *Frontiers in Neuroscience* 9 (January 1, 2015), https://doi.org/10.3389/fnins.2015.0 0225.
7. Linda Witek-Janusek, Sheryl Gabram, and Herbert L. Mathews, "Psychologic Stress, Reduced NK Cell Activity, and Cytokine Dysregulation in Women Experiencing Diagnostic Breast Biopsy," *Psychoneuroendocrinology* 32, no. 1 (January 1, 2007), https://doi.org/10.1016/j.psyneuen.2006.09.011.

67. Maximize the amount of nutrients per bite.

1. C. A Reider et al., "Inadequacy of Immune Health Nutrients: Intakes in US Adults, the 2005–2016 NHANES," *Nutrients* 12(6) (June 10, 2020): 1735, doi: 10.3390/nu12061735. PMID: 32531972; PMCID: PMC7352522.
2. J. C. Soares et al., "Preserving the Nutritional Quality of Crop Plants Under a Changing Climate: Importance and Strategies," *Plant and Soil* 443(1–2) (2019): 1–26, https://doi.org/10.1007/s11104-019-04229-0.
3. Stephan van Vliet, Frederick D. Provenza, and Scott L. Kronberg, "Health-Promoting Phytonutrients Are Higher in Grass-Fed Meat and Milk," *Frontiers in Sustainable Food Systems* 4 (February 1, 2021), https://doi.org/10.3389 /fsufs.2020.555426.

68. Floss (and tongue scrape!).

1. María Martínez et al., "The Role of the Oral Microbiota Related to Periodontal Diseases in Anxiety, Mood and Trauma- and Stress-Related Disorders," *Frontiers in Psychiatry* 12 (January 1, 2021), https://doi.org/10.3389/fpsyt .2021.814177.
2. Mireya Martínez-García and Enrique Hernández-Lemus, "Periodontal

Inflammation and Systemic Diseases: An Overview," *Frontiers in Physiology* 12 (January 1, 2021), https://doi.org/10.3389/fphys.2021.709438.

3. Leslie Borsa, Margaux Dubois, Guillaume Sacco, and Laurence Lupi, "Analysis the Link between Periodontal Diseases and Alzheimer's Disease: A Systematic Review," *International Journal of Environmental Research and Public Health* 18, no. 17 (September 1, 2021), https://doi.org/10.3390/ijerph18179312.

4. Shalini Kanagasingam et al., "Porphyromonas Gingivalis Is a Strong Risk Factor for Alzheimer's Disease," *Journal of Alzheimer's Disease Reports* 4, no. 1 (January 1, 2020), https://doi.org/10.3233/ADR-200250.

5. S. Asher et al., "Periodontal Health, Cognitive Decline, and Dementia: A Systematic Review and Meta-analysis of Longitudinal Studies," *Journal of the American Geriatrics Society* 70(9) (2022): 2695–2709, https://doi.org/10.1111/jgs.17978.

6. Trent L. Outhouse et al., "A Cochrane Systematic Review Finds Tongue Scrapers Have Short-Term Efficacy in Controlling Halitosis – PubMed," *General Dentistry* 54, no. 5 (October 1, 2006).

69. Stop snoring.

1. Apoor S. Gami et al., "Obstructive Sleep Apnea and the Risk of Sudden Cardiac Death: A Longitudinal Study of 10,701 Adults," *Journal of the American College of Cardiology* 62, no. 7 (August 13, 2013): 610–16, https://doi.org/10.1016/j.jacc.2013.04.080.

2. M. Ichioka et al., "Changes of Circulating Atrial Natriuretic Peptide and Antidiuretic Hormone in Obstructive Sleep Apnea Syndrome," *Respiration* 59(3) (1992): 164–68, doi:10.1159/000196049.

70. Upgrade the foods you're already eating.

1. M. Xia et al., "Olive Oil Consumption and Risk of Cardiovascular Disease and All-Cause Mortality: A Meta-analysis of Prospective Cohort Studies," *Frontiers in Nutrition* 9 (2022), https://doi.org/10.3389/fnut.2022.1041203.

2. J. F. Millman et al., "Extra-virgin Olive Oil and the Gut-Brain Axis: Influence on Gut Microbiota, Mucosal Immunity, and Cardiometabolic and Cognitive Health," *Nutrition Reviews*, 79(12) (2021): 1362–1374, https://doi.org/10.1093/nutrit/nuaa148.

3. Sylvie Lamy et al., "Olive Oil Compounds Inhibit Vascular Endothelial Growth Factor Receptor-2 Phosphorylation," *Experimental Cell Research* 322, no. 1 (March 10, 2014), https://doi.org/10.1016/j.yexcr.2013.11.022.

4. S. Bastida and F. J. Sánchez-Muniz, "Thermal Oxidation of Olive Oil, Sunflower Oil and a Mix of Both Oils during Forty Discontinuous Domestic Fryings of Different Foods," *Food Science and Technology International* 7, no. 1 (February 1, 2001): 15–21, https://doi.org/10.1177/108201301772662644.

5. Linus Pauling Institute, "Garlic," April 28, 2014, https://lpi.oregonstate.edu/mic/food-beverages/garlic.

6. Leyla Bayan, Peir Hossain Koulivand, and Ali Gorji, "Garlic: A Review of Potential Therapeutic Effects," *Avicenna Journal of Phytomedicine* 4, no. 1 (February 1, 2014).

7. Roman Leontiev et al., "A Comparison of the Antibacterial and Antifungal Activities of Thiosulfinate Analogues of Allicin," *Scientific Reports* 8, no. 1 (April 30, 2018): 1–19, https://doi.org/10.1038/s41598-018-25154-9.

8. Chuanhai Zhang et al., "Allicin-Induced Host-Gut Microbe Interactions Improves Energy Homeostasis," *FASEB Journal* 34, no. 8 (July 3, 2020): 10682–98, https://doi.org/10.1096/fj.202001007r.

9. Patrizia Riso et al., "DNA Damage and Repair Activity after Broccoli Intake in

Young Healthy Smokers," *Mutagenesis* 25, no. 6 (August 16, 2010): 595–602, https://doi.org/10.1093/mutage/geq045.

10. Patricia A. Egner et al., "Rapid and Sustainable Detoxication of Airborne Pollutants by Broccoli Sprout Beverage: Results of a Randomized Clinical Trial in China," *Cancer Prevention Research* 7, no. 8 (August 1, 2014): 813–23, https://doi.org/10.1158/1940-6207.capr-14-0103.

11. I. Sarvan et al., "Sulforaphane Formation and Bioaccessibility Are More Affected by Steaming Time than Meal Composition during in Vitro Digestion of Broccoli – PubMed," *Food Chemistry* 214 (January 1, 2017), https://doi.org/10.1016/j.foodchem.2016.07.111.

12. Khalil Ghawi, "The Potential to Intensify Sulforaphane Formation in Cooked Broccoli (*Brassica oleracea* var. *italica*) Using Mustard Seeds (*Sinapis alba*)," *Food Chemistry* 138, no. 2–3 (June 1, 2013): 1734–41, https://doi.org/10.1016/j.foodchem.2012.10.119.

71. Challenge limiting aging beliefs.

1. Becca R. Levy et al., "Longevity Increased by Positive Self-Perceptions of Aging," *Journal of Personality and Social Psychology* 83, no. 2 (August 1, 2002), https://doi.org/10.1037//0022-3514.83.2.261.

72. Reassess your relationship with alcohol.

1. "Chronic Disease Fact Sheet: Cancer," Centers for Disease Control, June 7, 2022, https://www.cdc.gov/chronicdisease/resources/publications/factsheets/cancer.htm.

2. Dipak Sarkar, M. Katherine Jung, and H. Joe Wang, "Alcohol and the Immune System," *Alcohol Research: Current Reviews* 37, no. 2 (January 1, 2015).

3. Juan I. Garaycoechea et al., "Alcohol and Endogenous Aldehydes Damage Chromosomes and Mutate Stem Cells," *Nature* 553, no. 7687 (January 3, 2018): 171–77, https://doi.org/10.1038/nature25154.

4. J. Pan et al., "Alcohol Consumption and the Risk of Gastroesophageal Reflux Disease: A Systematic Review and Meta-analysis," *Alcohol and Alcoholism* 54(1) (2019): 62–69, doi: 10.1093/alcalc/agy063.

5. L. T. Crow, "Diencephalic Influence in Alcohol Diuresis," *Physiology & Behavior* 3 (1968): 319–22, doi: 10.1016/0031-9384(68)90107-8.

6. Mahesh M. Thakkar, Rishi Sharma, and Pradeep Sahota, "Alcohol Disrupts Sleep Homeostasis," *Alcohol* 49, no. 4 (June 1, 2015), https://doi.org/10.1016/j.alcohol.2014.07.019.

7. E. Baraona and C. S. Lieber, "Effects of Ethanol on Lipid Metabolism – PubMed," *Journal of Lipid Research* 20, no. 3 (March 1, 1979).

8. Niladri Banerjee, "Neurotransmitters in Alcoholism: A Review of Neurobiological and Genetic Studies," *Indian Journal of Human Genetics* 20, no. 1 (March 1, 2014), https://doi.org/10.4103/0971-6866.132750.

9. World Health Organization, "Alcohol Is One of the Biggest Risk Factors for Breast Cancer," *World Health Organization: WHO*, October 20, 2021, https://www.who.int/europe/news/item/20-10-2021-alcohol-is-one-of-the-biggest-risk-factors-for-breast-cancer.

75. Meditate—but for less time than you think.

1. M. De Couck et al., "How Breathing Can Help You Make Better Decisions: Two Studies on the Effects of Breathing Patterns on Heart Rate Variability and Decision-making in Business Cases," *International Journal of Psychophysiology* 139 (2019): 1–9, doi:10.1016/j.ijpsycho.2019.02.011.

77. Stop letting fear control your relationship with money.

1. "Newsroom | Northwestern Mutual," 2018, https://news.northwesternmutual.com/planning-and-progress-2018.

79. Try a breathwork practice.

1. Melis Yilmaz Balban et al., "Brief Structured Respiration Practices Enhance Mood and Reduce Physiological Arousal," *Cell Reports Medicine* 4, no. 1 (January 17, 2023), https://doi.org/10.1016/j.xcrm.2022.100895.
2. Melis Yilmaz Balban et al., "Brief Structured Respiration Practices Enhance Mood and Reduce Physiological Arousal," *Cell Reports Medicine* 4, no. 1 (January 2023): 100895, https://doi.org/10.1016/j.xcrm.2022.100895.

81. Give your brain a bath.

1. Nina Markil et al., "Yoga Nidra Relaxation Increases Heart Rate Variability and Is Unaffected by a Prior Bout of Hatha Yoga – PubMed," *Journal of Alternative and Complementary Medicine* 18, no. 10 (October 1, 2012), https://doi.org/10.1089/acm.2011.0331.
2. Esther N. Moszeik, Timo von Oertzen, and Karl-Heinz Renner, "Effectiveness of a Short Yoga Nidra Meditation on Stress, Sleep, and Well-Being in a Large and Diverse Sample," *Current Psychology* 41, no. 8 (September 8, 2020): 5272–86, https://doi.org/10.1007/s12144-020-01042-2.

83. Utilize the healing power of nature.

1. Jesper J. Alvarsson, Stefan Wiens, and Mats E. Nilsson, "Stress Recovery during Exposure to Nature Sound and Environmental Noise," *International Journal of Environmental Research and Public Health* 7, no. 3 (March 1, 2010), https://doi.org/10.3390/ijerph7031036.
2. H. Jo, C. Song, and Y. Miyazaki, "Physiological Benefits of Viewing Nature: A Systematic Review of Indoor Experiments," *International Journal of Environmental Research and Public Health* 16(23) (November 27, 2019): 4739, doi: 10.3390/ijerph16234739. PMID: 31783531; PMCID: PMC6926748.
3. Kate Lee, "40-Second Green Roof Views Sustain Attention: The Role of Micro-Breaks in Attention Restoration," *Journal of Environmental Psychology* 42 (June 2015): 182–89, https://doi.org/10.1016/j.jenvp.2015.04.003.
4. R. S. Ulrich, "View through a Window May Influence Recovery from Surgery," *Science* 224, no. 4647 (April 27, 1984), https://doi.org/10.1126/science.6143402.
5. Jesper J. Alvarsson, Stefan Wiens, and Mats E. Nilsson, "Stress Recovery during Exposure to Nature Sound and Environmental Noise," *International Journal of Environmental Research and Public Health* 7, no. 3 (March 1, 2010), https://doi.org/10.3390/ijerph7031036.
6. Q. Li et al., "Visiting a Forest, but Not a City, Increases Human Natural Killer Activity and Expression of Anti-Cancer Proteins," *International Journal of Immunopathology and Pharmacology* 21, no. 1 (January 2008): 117–27, https://doi.org/10.1177/039463200802100113.
7. Jessica M. Yano et al., "Indigenous Bacteria from the Gut Microbiota Regulate Host Serotonin Biosynthesis," *Cell* 161, no. 2 (April 9, 2015), https://doi.org/10.1016/j.cell.2015.02.047.

86. Tap into the intelligence of your body.

1. Narayanan Kandasamy et al., "Interoceptive Ability Predicts Survival on a London Trading Floor," *Scientific Reports* 6, no. 1 (September 19, 2016): 1–7, https://doi.org/10.1038/srep32986.

88. Get specific with your emotions.

1.   H. M. Lefcourt, "The Humor Solution," in C. R. Snyder (ed.), *Coping with Stress: Effective People and Processes* (London: Oxford University Press, 2001), 68–92.
2.   M. M. Tugade and B. L. Fredrickson, "Resilient Individuals Use Positive Emotions to Bounce Back from Negative Emotional Experiences," *Journal of Personality and Social Psychology* 86 (2004): 320–33.

89. Have no regrets when you die.

1.   C. Saffrey, A. Summerville, and N. J. Roese, "Praise for Regret: People Value Regret above Other Negative Emotions," *Motivation and Emotion* 32(1) (March 2008): 46–54, doi: 10.1007/s11031-008-9082-4. PMID: 18535665; PMCID: PMC2413060.
2.   J. Reb, "Regret Aversion and Decision Process Quality: Effects of Regret Salience on Decision Process Carefulness," *Organizational Behavior and Human Decision Processes* 105(2) (2008): 169–82, https://doi.org/10.1016/j.obhdp.2007.08.006.
3.   E. Kross and O. Ayduk, "Making Meaning Out of Negative Experiences by Self-distancing," *Current Directions in Psychological Science* 20(3) (2011): 187–91, https://doi.org/10.1177/0963721411408883.

98. Get to the root of low libido.

1.   Kevin Lewandowski, T. Schrage, and L. Caya, "A Comparison of Relationship Satisfaction and Sexual Satisfaction in Short-Term and Long-Term Relationships," *Psychology*, 2010.

99. Reduce your pain.

1.   Asma Hayati Ahmad and Rahimah Zakaria, "Pain in Times of Stress," *Malaysian Journal of Medical Sciences* 22, Special Issue (December 1, 2015).

About the Author

Liz Moody is the host of the top-rated *The Liz Moody Podcast*, where, alongside her world-class expert guests, she shares actionable, research-backed advice about gut health, hormone health, longevity, finances, relationships, mental health, and more—anything and everything that helps people live their healthiest, happiest lives.

Liz is also the bestselling author of *Healthier Together: Recipes for Two—Nourish Your Body, Nourish Your Relationships* and *Glow Pops*, a former nationally syndicated newspaper columnist, and a decades-long journalist for publications like *Marie Claire*, goop, and mindbodygreen, a leading wellness website where she led the content strategy for the food section and later served as editor-at-large.

With millions of community members across her podcast and social media, Liz has built a reputation as a trusted resource who makes science-backed tips and tools fun, accessible, and interesting. A graduate of UC Berkeley, she lives nomadically with her husband, Zack, and cat, Bella.

You can find more tips like the ones in this book on *The Liz Moody Podcast*, available on all podcast platforms, and on her social media @lizmoody on Instagram and TikTok.